Research in Criminology

Series Editors
Alfred Blumstein
David P. Farrington

Research in Criminology

Edward Zamble
Frank J. Porporino

Coping, Behavior, and Adaptation in Prison Inmates

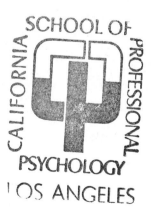

Springer-Verlag
New York Berlin Heidelberg
London Paris Tokyo

Edward Zamble
Department of Psychology, Queen's University, Kingston, Ontario
K7L 3N6, Canada

Frank J. Porporino
Ministry of the Solicitor General of Canada, Ottawa, Ontario
K1S 2C3 Canada

Series Editors
Alfred Blumstein
School of Urban and Public Affairs, Carnegie-Mellon University,
Pittsburgh, Pennsylvania 15213, USA

David P. Farrington
Institute of Criminology, University of Cambridge, Cambridge CB3 9DT, England

Library of Congress Cataloging-in-Publication Data
Zamble, Edward.
  Coping, behavior, and adaptation in prison inmates/by Edward
Zamble and Frank Porporino.
    p.   cm.—(Research in criminology)
  Bibliography: p.
  Includes index.
  ISBN 0-387-96613-7
  1. Prison psychology—Case studies.   2. Adjustment (Psychology)—
Case studies.   I. Porporino, Frank.   II. Title.   III. Series.
HV6089.Z36   1988
365'.6'019—dc 19   87-33097
                                                                          CIP

Typeset by Asco Trade Typesetting Ltd., Hong Kong.
Printed and bound by R.R. Donnelley & Sons, Harrisonburg, Virginia.
Printed in the United States of America.

9 8 7 6 5 4 3 2 1

ISBN 0-387-96613-7 Springer-Verlag New York Berlin Heidelberg
ISBN 3-540-96613-7 Springer-Verlag Berlin Heidelberg New York

This book is dedicated to all those on both sides of the barriers who have to cope everyday with the reality of prison life

Preface

This book is the report of a collaborative effort. Frank Porporino and I arrived at the starting point for our work together by very different routes. Originally trained as an experimental psychologist, I had become increasingly restive within the confines of the laboratory, and spent a sabbatical year in the equivalent of a clinical internship. I then spent some time as a part-time consultant in a local penitentiary.

Most of my time in the institution was spent with inmates with a variety of problems, probably about 50 individuals over the course of a year. Although this was far fewer than a full-time psychologist in the system might encounter, it served as a quick cram course on problem prisoners and prisoner problems. Very quickly my stereotypes about convicts were shown to be virtually useless. I learned that the criminal classes included all levels of society, and that the behavior of prisoners was the same as that of other human beings in a difficult environment.

My preconceptions about the destructive effects of imprisonment had been reinforced by the obvious unpleasantness of the environment, so I expected to find many men who were functionally disabled, but this was not what I saw. Of course my prison "clients" were almost all having trouble dealing with life. This was not surprising, for they would not have been referred to me if they were perfectly adapted and content with their circumstances. At the same time, they were very different from the more passive inmates I had seen in other types of institutions, for most of them seemed to be actively trying to deal with their problems. Indeed, I was impressed with the energy with which many of them struggled, but often I had the image of a fish on a hook: the harder it struggles, the worse things become.

It struck me that in many ways their behavior was similar to that portrayed in the literature on the training of coping skills. Thus, I was led to abandon prior notions and to the idea that many prison inmates have inadequate coping skills. I thought that their deficiencies might be linked to some of their problems in prison.

At about this time, I had begun speaking to Frank about the possibility of supervising his Ph.D. thesis. He had come to Queen's University with an M.A. in clinical psychology, with particular expertise in psychometric methods. He had also worked for several years on the front lines as a psychologist in a federal penitentiary. When I tried to tell Frank about my new ideas, I discovered that he had been thinking along the same lines. After a few discussions, we shaped each other's thoughts until we agreed on the potential usefulness of coping theory in dealing with prisoner behavior, and we decided to attempt some systematic research on the subject.

The result is a story of a little study that grew. We realized that we needed some financial and political support in order to carry out the research, so we spoke with people in the Research Division of the Solicitor General in Ottawa. We were encouraged to make a formal proposal. Of course, this meant that we had to work out procedures and measures, so we spent close to a year in the preliminary stage. There was also a lot of waiting for clearances, permissions, and signatures. The longer it took, the more we wanted to make the work definitive, for we were not sure we would ever get a second chance, or would want to fight through the process again. So the study grew and grew, but we hope it is better as a result.

At the time of this writing, it has been over eight years since our original letters of intent. In the interim, Frank finished his thesis on a project closely related to our principal line of research (but not included here) and moved on to the Ministry of the Solicitor General in Ottawa. By now, we have been through so many discussions that neither of us knows who originated any specific idea. We have also gone through so many stages of the written report that it would take a stylistic analysis by a sophisticated computer program to disentangle our separate contributions.

During the course of this study, we had a wide range of experiences, from the drama and shock of an assistant taken hostage, to moments of bathos and low comedy in some of our interviews with subjects. (Imagine, for example, an interviewer and an inmate locked in a room together when the lock breaks; after the guards make emergency calls for tools to take the door out of the frame, the inmate calmly finishes the discussion and then picks the lock.) However, these are perhaps best told in other places, perhaps in the play I keep threatening to write.

We are grateful to the many people without whose efforts this work could not have been done—or done as well. Naming them all would fill several pages. However, we must single out Julia Kalotay who was the principal research assistant for most of the study. She conducted the majority of the actual interviews; undoubtedly her sensitive and sympathetic questioning was a major factor in maintaining the level of cooperation we got from both subjects and institutional staff.

We are also grateful to the Research Division of the Solicitor General of Canada for both material and personal support. Hugh Haley encouraged us at the beginning, John Evans helped us through the rough spots, and

Helen Durie was indispensable at all stages. Their vision and support were often beyond the call of duty, and without them we could not have accomplished anything.

In our presentation of the study, we have worked to strike a balance. On the one hand, we have tried to objectify and quantify things rigorously in the data and in its analyses; as scientists, we could do no less. On the other hand, we have also tried to remember that behind the statistical agglomerates and analyses, we were dealing with real people in real situations; as psychologists, this is our responsibility. From either side, the things we found were often discrepant with our expectations or desires, but we have done our best to convey an accurate picture of the reality we found rather than our preconceptions. We hope that the reader will judge our efforts to be not entirely unsuccessful.

Kingston, Ontario   Edward Zamble
July 1987

Contents

Contents

No mind is much employed upon the present; recollection and anticipation fill up almost all our moments.

—Samuel Johnson

The past is dead. If I think about it, it will kill me too.

—Inmate subject X

How often do I think about the future? If I get through this day, I have 5,000 more exactly like it ahead of me. I just try to survive each hour.

—Inmate subject Y

1
Introduction

Corrections has changed in significant ways over the past several decades. Prisons have become less militaristic, more humane, and somewhat less insular. For the most part, they have been transformed into institutions that function under the rules of procedure, administrative policies, and organizational cultures of complex, street-level bureaucracies (Lipsky, 1980).

Corrections, in one sense, has progressed. It has moved to become more mindful of the rights of offenders, the concerns of staff, and the expectations of the public. In other ways, however, it has remained riddled with problems so severe as to challenge the very meaningfulness of the entire enterprise.

In the past decade or so we have witnessed growing fear of crime and a swing towards more punitive, retributive, and intolerant public attitudes. The criminal justice system has responded in kind. Rates of imprisonment have been rising in many Western countries, and in some places they have reached an all-time high (Austin and Krisberg, 1985; Gottfredson, 1986). For example, it has been estimated that one out of every 35 adult American males is currently under some form of criminal justice restraint (Gottfredson, 1986). At current rates, one out of every 20 males born in the United States can be expected to serve a term in a state prison (Bureau of Justice Statistics, 1985). Despite an unprecedented increase in prison construction, resources have been strained to the limit, and prison crowding may have become the predominant and pervasive correctional problem of the decade (Blumstein, 1986; Garry, 1984; Gottfredson and McConville, 1986).

The character of correctional populations has also changed substantially. Prisons must now manage a more diverse group of offenders serving longer prison terms for a wider range of offences. They must contend with greater concentrations of mentally disordered offenders, drug and alcohol abusers, young violent offenders, racial and ethnic minorities, and, especially, offenders with histories of serious violent acts.

With all of this to confront, debate as to the proper role and aims of imprisonment as a means of crime control has left corrections in a state of uncertainty and ambivalence regarding its mission. Correctional staff and administrators often feel frustrated and demoralized by the confusing diversity of demands on the system and the variety of conflicting goals that they are often asked to implement. Perhaps as a result, they remain focused on the daily functioning of their institutions, with the persistent need to maintain order and control despite a never-ending stream of operational crises and chronic shortages of resources.

In short, corrections has evolved to where it is pulled rather than driven. Observers and students of the prison have continued in their attempts to clarify purpose (Cullen and Gilbert, 1982; Johnson, 1987; Thomas, 1987). Yet the effect on correctional policy and practice seems minimal. Reforms may be contemplated, but the persistence and vision needed to pursue them vigorously seem to be lacking.

We believe that one reason for this situation is that the knowledge as to how to redirect corrections is also lacking. In order to be sound and reasonable, the design and operation of prisons should be based not on any particular theory or ideology, but on some fundamental understanding of how imprisonment affects individuals. The clarification of the mission for the correctional system must begin with a valid and verifiable appreciation of how imprisonment impinges on human beings: whether it damages or leaves them intact; whether it affects some and not others; whether it affects people only in some ways or under particular circumstances.

The question of how imprisonment affects individuals has concerned social scientists for over half a century. In the face of more complex and more pressing problems in the correctional system, the question becomes even more important. Corrections will likely remain troubled and confused until we understand more clearly how imprisonment affects prisoners.

This book is concerned with the behavior of men in prison. At some points it reaches farther and touches on aspects of a theory to explain much of criminal behavior, but it centers on what prisoners do under the conditions of contemporary confinement, how they approach their lives, and how they adapt to the problems and difficulties they experience. In subsequent chapters we will describe the methods, results, and implications of a major-scale empirical study that examines these issues. However, before we proceed to the study this chapter will consider the background of the ideas involved and will attempt to explain the theoretical perspective from which the work derives.

Theory and Context: Understanding the Causes of Behavior

Western thought about the nature of the forces that shape human behavior has been essentially bifurcated for several centuries. On one hand is the assumption that the wellsprings of our actions are within us. On the other side is the view that we are shaped by our external environment.

While we are oversimplifying the distinction here for heuristic purposes, one cannot overestimate the importance of this division into two kinds of explanation. The controversy between the two paths has dominated the development of ideas for generations of theorists in a variety of fields. We may see the conflict between the ideologies of capitalism and communism as one example of how the contrasting explanations of behavior can inspire deep philosophical and political differences. Clearly, the rift of difference between these two approaches in accounting for behavior can be wide and deep.

In the universe of psychological problems, the difference is embodied in the historical controversy between environmentalists and nativists or personality theorists (Mischel, 1973). The former, most radically personified by extreme Watsonian behaviorists, argue that external events and contingencies can overwhelm all other determinants and force behavior into predictable and uniform patterns. Individual differences may be explained as the result of differing environmental histories, and failures of prediction can be rationalized as the fault of insufficiently powerful contingencies.

In contrast, many other theorists have attempted to show how a variety of internal mechanisms may be used to explain or predict actions. These include everything from global personality constructs of overriding theoretical importance to controllers of minor responses. They include explanations of universal behavior, usually seen as the inevitable expression of shared genetic material or the result of universal personality archetypes, and also of individual differences, seen as the result of variety in genetic or other internal structures. All these explanations have in common the expectation that behavior can best be understood as the result of consistent and enduring internal structures.

The conflict between adherents of these two opposing viewpoints has been renewed episodically over the history of modern psychology. The resulting interchanges have been often vehement, sometimes bitter, and ultimately probably fruitless. For despite the temptations of slogans, such as the catchphrase reducing the controversy to "nature versus nurture," as is usually the case in polarized conflicts the debate has over the decades generated more heat than light.

This may, of course, have occurred because the details of the correct position are yet to be worked out, as adherents customarily claim, but we believe rather that it is because the reality of behavior resists the simplifications of either side. In their insistence on the ultimate sensibleness of either model, the great majority of theorists have ignored the interaction of internal and external determinants. Very few models have considered how specified aspects of the environment will affect individuals with differing behavioral propensities, or how individuals with particular personal characteristics will react to variation in external conditions and situations.

In a few cases, we expect that behavior will be uniquely determined by environmental conditions. For example, a total lack of food ought to lead to some sort of food-seeking behavior in every intact individual. Similarly, we can predict that some internal characteristics will have inevitable results on actions. For example, we can predict that a blind person will fail to react to any purely visual cues.

However, when we study the range of situations that commonly occur in our lives, we can conclude that there are few internal dispositions that are so powerful as to uniquely determine actions in all situations, and few environmental events that can compel identical responses from people of every disposition. In general, we would expect that the interaction between individuals and situations will be the most powerful predictor of behavior.

Interaction and Action

While the debate between internal and external theorists of behavior has employed many arguments, we believe that in the end both extremes are incorrect. While each has some evidence to support it, each is wrong in denying the influence of other factors. The most sensible answer comes from a synthesis that recognizes the evidence on both sides. In some ways, both sides are wrong, both are right, and the answer lies somewhere else. We can see that neither viewpoint alone can provide adequate explanations or predictions of behavior.

Take first the environmentalist approach. We can recognize that external events can have some very powerful effect on behavior, for example through conditioning and motivational or reinforcement processes. In an infant these may have powerful effects on observed behavior. However, we know that environments differ across individuals, and also across time for the same individual. If we believe that the environment leaves its effect, then after an accumulation of experiences the way a person reacts to his environment will be altered.

It matters not that this is caused by the action of external forces: the end result is that we cannot predict actions from knowledge of local conditions alone. Eventually, the accumulation of experience produces individual differences in ways of responding, and an understanding of behavior requires that these be taken into account. In effect, even a strictly environmentalist position requires that "personality" be taken into account, even if it is originally created by the action of external factors.

Similarly, even the strictest personality theorist must agree that the consequences of our actions have some internal representation. Even if action is determined by strong internal propensities, memories of past actions will be taken into account in determining new actions. No reasonable theorist would argue that behavior is invariant regardless of circumstances, and this implies that the external situation must be represented internally.

If this is so, even if the effects of the environment are represented in ways determined by individual personality patterns, such effects must be considered in order to make any sensible predictions about behavior. Thus, when one deals with a mature individual the effects of experience must be considered, regardless of the original source of the actions which comprise that experience.

These arguments lead us to the position that in the end the differences between the two schools of thought are moot. Regardless of which side one starts from, it must always be acknowledged that behavior results from an interaction of both internal and external factors. The general debate about which side is correct reduces to consideration of the specific factors entering into the control or evocation of specific actions at particular times and under specified circumstances. We believe that most of the interesting variance in behavior lies in the interaction between internal and environmental factors, and a century of debate between extreme positions has served only to obscure this fact.

In the work to be described in this book, we wanted to deal with the behavior of men in prison. Our particular interest was to understand how prisons affect individuals and, conversely, how individuals function to shape their prison experiences. Our approach was grounded in an interactionist model of the causes of human behavior (Bowers, 1973; Lazarus and Folkman, 1983; Magnussen and Endler, 1977). Therefore, we decided that we must study not just the conditions and situations that arise during imprisonment but also how individual offenders come to perceive these conditions, react to situations, and behave differently as their term progresses.

We did not suppose, as others have done before us, that the pains of imprisonment would have inevitable effects on behavior (Goffman, 1961; Johnson and Toch, 1982; Sykes, 1958). Similarly, we did not expect that the characteristics and dispositions of offenders on admission would be so predominant as to determine behavior across conditions or situations of confinement (Clemmer, 1958; Irwin and Cressey, 1962). We set out to find evidence for a more underlying process that would tell us how external and internal factors might interact in determining different kinds of reactions to imprisonment.

The part of the process that we chose to study is the subject of contemporary psychological theories about how humans respond to, or cope with, stressful life circumstances. We will elaborate the model later in this chapter. Suffice it to say at this point that we set out to operationalize our interactionist perspective by examining the appraisals and coping behaviors that appear as offenders negotiate their time in prison.

To summarize our perspective here, we begin from the assumption that the determinants of real behavior are complex, multiple, and interactive. This applies to the behavior of prisoners as well as to that of other individuals in other circumstances. Actions can be explained only by considering both the situation and the ways of reacting that a person brings to that situation.

The emphasis on the interaction between persons and events is far from unique here. Indeed, it is arguably becoming the predominant point of view in contemporary psychology. It should be noted that the change has seemed to accompany the rebirth of interest in the nature and role of cognitions among academic research psychologists (Estes, 1975). Perhaps this is because interactions are so readily apparent in cognitive processes, or perhaps it is because the demonstration of the usefulness of interactionist thinking in cognitions provides a good concrete example of how such thinking can be extended to other sorts of behavior.

In any case, the position argued here is but one example of a general trend in contemporary experimental and clinical psychology. Moreover, there are indications that even this is only part of a more general trend, and that similar ideas are also having their effect in other areas. For example, Cullen (1983) presents an argument for a restructuring of deviance theory in sociology. Although his terms are different, it is readily apparent that the direction of his thinking is entirely parallel to ours.

In general, however, theory and research in psychology has had only a minimal impact on criminology. The mainstream of criminology, for the most part, seems to have ignored the application of cognitive and social learning principles for explaining offender behavior. (There are a few exceptions: for example, see Little and Kendall, 1979; Ross and Fabiano, 1985.) This seems to be particularly true in the area of corrections, where the forces that account for the behavior of prisoners during confinement have befuddled criminologists for decades.

Before we proceed with a more detailed explanation of our coping model for behavior, it is appropriate here to review previous research on the effects of imprisonment. This literature spans the fields of sociology, psychology, and psychiatry. It has been reviewed in considerable depth elsewhere (e.g., Bonta and Gendreau, 1987; Bowker, 1977; Bukstel and Kilmann, 1980; McKay, Jayewardene, and Reedie, 1977; Thomas and Petersen, 1977; Walker, 1983; Wormith, 1984a). Therefore, our purpose here is only to consider where this research has brought us, and, in particular, to highlight its methodological and conceptual deficiencies. We shall see that studies in the area have failed to advance our understanding a great deal, and we will argue that this is principally because they have ignored the need for interactionist thinking or methodologies.

We should also mention that some autobiographical and qualitatively based accounts of the prison experience have provided rich and compelling descriptions of how prisoners cope (e.g., Abbott, 1981; Alper, 1974; Caron, 1978; Clayton, 1970; Cohen and Taylor, 1972; Manocchio and Dunn, 1970; Pell, 1972). While we acknowledge the value of some of the ideas in this work, we must admit that it served to reinforce our interests but not to guide our thinking. Our reviewing of the area focuses on the empirical literature.

Sociological Analyses of Imprisonment

The sociological literature on imprisonment is dominated by what are fairly dated analyses of prisoners' adoption of subculture norms, attitudes, and various institutional argot roles. Early field studies detailed the emergence of an informal social world within the prison environment, one with its own unique social classes, language, economy, and rules governing behavior (Clemmer, 1958; Garabedian, 1963; Irwin and Cressey, 1962; Morris and Morris, 1963; Schrag, 1954; Sykes, 1958; Sykes and Messinger, 1960).

From the functional or systems perspective which was then emerging within sociological theory, the social control processes in the prison were regarded as having a profound and direct influence on the behavior of all inmates. These processes were seen as representing the central collective solution to the peculiar problems and "pains of imprisonment." The dynamics of assimilation into the prison culture, summarized by Clemmer with the term *prisonization*, have since preoccupied sociological research and theory on the prison experience.

Until recently, the research has followed two competing hypotheses, summarized as the deprivation and importation models of prisonization (Thomas and Petersen, 1977). The deprivation model emphasizes intra-institutional pressures and problems generated by the actual experience of imprisonment (Sykes, 1958; Sykes and Messinger, 1960). Prisonization is seen as the consequence of "depersonalizing and stigmatizing effects of legal processing and induction into the prison, coupled with the alienative effects of the coercive power exercised by prison officials in their attempts to maintain social control within the prison" (Thomas, 1977, p. 137).

Studies based on the deprivation model have examined the relationships between prisonization and a variety of factors, including: (a) the length of time in prison and the time remaining to be served (Akers, Hayner, and Gruninger, 1977; Atchley and McCabe, 1968; Clemmer, 1950; Wellford, 1967; Wheeler, 1961); (b) interpersonal involvements and the social role assumed by the inmate (Garabedian, 1964; Schrag, 1961; Sykes and Messinger, 1960); (c) the type of institution and organizational structure (Akers et al., 1977; Berk, 1966; Cline, 1968; Street, 1965); and (d) the degree of alienation or powerlessness experienced by the inmate (Thomas and Poole, 1975; Thomas and Zingraff, 1976; Tittle and Tittle, 1964).

The deprivation model's closed-system emphasis on prison-specific influences is challenged by the importation model. Importation theory highlights the effects that preprison socialization and experience can have on adaptation to prison life. Within the importation model, the degree and

duration of involvement with criminal value systems prior to imprisonment, and the various attitudinal and behavioral patterns that the inmate
brings with him to prison are regarded as the most crucial determinants of
adaptation (Irwin, 1970; Irwin and Cressey, 1962; Thomas and Petersen,
1977).

Preprison factors that have been related to prisonization include: (a)
general social history factors such as age, race, educational attainment, and
preoffense socioeconomic and employment status (Alpert, 1979; Jensen
and Jones, 1976; Schwartz, 1971; Thomas, 1977); (b) variables reflecting
the individual's history of criminal involvement, such as the number of
prior convictions and the number and length of prior prison terms (Alpert,
1979; Wellford, 1967; Zingraff, 1980); (c) identification with criminal
values and attitudes toward the legal system (Thomas and Poole, 1975;
Zingraff, 1980); (d) the self-concept of the individual (Faine, 1973; Hepburn and Stratton, 1977; Tittle, 1972); and (e) identification with broad
social, political, racial, and religious ideologies (Irwin, 1980; Jacobs, 1976).

Given the amount of research on both varieties of prisonization theory,
the results have been disappointing. The theoretical linkages made between
prisonization and various intrainstitutional or preprison predisposing
factors have not been borne out. Only weak and inconsistent relationships have been found (Bowker, 1977; Hawkins, 1976; Thomas, 1977;
Thomas and Petersen, 1977; Zingraff, 1980). Moreover, the hypothesized
associations with sentence phase have not been clarified, with discrepant
patterns emerging across studies (Atchley and McCabe, 1968; Bukstel and
Kilmann, 1980; Thomas, Petersen, and Zingraff, 1978; Troyer and Frease,
1975; Wheeler, 1961)

The meaningfulness of the prisonization construct is made even more
questionable by other findings. Although prisonization has been consistently related theoretically with decreased likelihood of postrelease
success, several studies have found an opposite relationship. Inmates who
subscribe to the inmate code and adjust poorly to the formal prison structure have been found to be less likely to be recidivists in comparison to their
less prisonized peers (Jaman, 1971; Kassebaum, Ward, and Wilner, 1971;
Miller and Dinitz, 1973). Other studies have shown that rebellious prisoners who reject formal prison rules and regulations are less handicapped
during the initial period of transition to the community (Goodstein, 1979)
and are actually more similar to "normal" persons outside prison on various
personality dimensions (Driscoll, 1952).

There is also considerable evidence that racial and cultural differences
exert a more powerful influence on behavior than the prescriptions of
the prison culture (Johnson, 1976). Indeed, the very existence of a stable
prison subculture and dominant convict identity has been disputed, a ten-
tative order based on values of violence and self-protection being seen as
having replaced the traditional prison social world (Irwin, 1980).

In summary, it is evident that prisonization has not served to clarify why and how prisoners adapt in particular ways during confinement. In view of the conceptual simplicity of the concept, this is not surprising. More recent studies have sought to integrate the deprivation and importation models, examining the predictive power of various combinations of factors (Thomas, 1977; Zingraff, 1980). However, the singular focus on prisonization as an explanatory construct has persisted.

There are several reasons for the lack of significant progress in understanding adaptation to imprisonment from the perspective of prisonization. Methodologically, the studies can be criticized for using different indices of prisonization, of unknown reliability and uncertain meaning (e.g., nonconformity with staff expectations, commitment to inmate solidarity, adherence to prescriptions of the inmate culture; cf. Poole, Regoli, and Thomas, 1980). There has also been a paucity of longitudinal analyses, most studies having relied on simple correlational or cross-sectional designs (Alpert, 1979). As we will consider in the next chapter, this limits what can correctly be concluded about changes over time (cf. Farrington, Ohlin, and Wilson, 1986).

However, the problems are more than just methodological. Although possibly of some heuristic value as a description of how imprisonment affects individuals, prisonization is clearly too general and too crude a construct. It has directed criminological research to the explanation of uniformity in behavior, rather than individual variation. Prison environments will affect individuals in myriad ways, and it is quite possible that individuals who become similarly "prisonized" will nonetheless vary on other dimensions determining important differences in adaptive functioning.

In order to understand varying reactions to imprisonment, a much finer analysis is needed than is afforded by the notion of prisonization. Using either deprivation or importation variables, studies that have looked at more specific aspects of behavior in prison have been much more successful than others in explaining observed variation in the behavior of inmates (e.g., Gibbs et al., 1985; Poole and Regoli, 1983; Toch, 1975, 1977). Rather than thinking of prisonization as a primary mode of adaptation to be predicted, it might be more useful if it were seen as an attitudinal factor that combines with other variables to affect adaptation.

Psychological Effects of Imprisonment

Studies that have sought to quantify the range of emotional or personality changes brought about by imprisonment are relatively more recent, even if they are not as numerous as those in the prisonization literature. However, once again, particular methodological and conceptual weaknesses have led to a set of inconsistent findings that are difficult to interpret.

Clinically and psychiatrically oriented case studies have long suggested that imprisonment can be devastating, at least for some offenders. For example, variants of a functional "psycho-syndrome" have been described which include defects in cognitive functioning (e.g., loss of memory and a general clouding of comprehension and ability to think), emotional problems (e.g., apathy and rigidity), problems in relating to others (e.g., infantile regression and increased introversion), and the appearance of various psychotic characteristics (e.g., obsessions, loss of reality contact; cf., Shorer, 1965; Heather, 1977). On the other hand, as one turns to studies that have applied more rigorous methodology, it becomes evident that there are no consistent findings of quantifiable psychological deterioration.

There have been numerous attempts to use traditional objective psychological measures to assess the effects of imprisonment. The MMPI has perhaps been used most extensively to determine how imprisonment may affect personality functioning. No clear conclusions can be derived from this literature (Gearing, 1979).

For our purposes, the work on the construct of self-esteem provides a good example of the inconsistencies that are found in other areas as well. Self-esteem has been a popular personality dimension to examine. Comparisons of findings are made difficult by differences in measures, subject sampling, and the time periods examined, and it is clear that no consensus of findings has emerged (Bukstel and Kilmann, 1980). For example, self-esteem has been found to increase after some period of imprisonment (Bennett, 1974; Gendreau, Gibson, Surridge and Hug, 1973), decrease (Fichtler, Zimmermann, and Moore, 1973; Hepburn and Stratton, 1977), or remain unchanged (Atchley and McCabe, 1968; Culbertson, 1975). Similar contradictory findings have been obtained with measures of other dimensions of psychological functioning.

Several studies have attempted to assess the effects of imprisonment using comprehensive batteries of psychological measures with groups of prisoners who varied in the amount of time they had served. The most well known of these is the series of studies carried out in England by a team of psychologists from Durham University (Banister, Smith, Heskin, and Bolton, 1973; Bolton, Smith, Heskin, and Banister, 1976; Heskin, Bolton, Smith, and Banister, 1974; Heskin, Smith, Banister, and Bolton, 1973).

The Durham group conducted a cross-sectional sampling of 175 prisoners who had been sentenced to long terms of imprisonment, with four groups varying in the amount of time served, from a mean of 2.5 years to a mean of 11.3 years. A subgroup of these prisoners was retested about 18 months later (Bolton et al., 1976). It was concluded that there was no overall deterioration in perceptual-motor or cognitive functioning associated with duration of imprisonment. Further, there were no consistent changes in attitudes or personality functioning attributable to the length of imprisonment.

Similar cross-sectional studies have been conducted in the Federal

Republic of Germany (Rasch, 1977, 1981), in England (Sapsford, 1978, 1983), and in Canada (Wormith, 1984b). Although Rasch noted that a large proportion of the prisoners he assessed showed signs of depression and emotional withdrawal, very few differences were found that covaried with the length of imprisonment. Furthermore, bitterness and expressions of demoralization by the prison environment (e.g., reports of sleep disturbance and loss of appetite) were most evident in the group of prisoners who had served the least time. This same pattern of greater distress in prisoners who had served less time was also observed by Sapsford (1978) on measures of anxiety, depression, and hopelessness.

Wormith (1984b) reported the findings from a battery of questionnaire measures administered to 269 Canadian federal offenders who had served from 1 month to 10 years. Controlling statistically for sentence length, age, and race, he found that time served covaried with significant improvement rather than deterioration on various measures of psychopathology, attitude, and personality.

Looking at the impact of imprisonment on a sample of long-term offenders in several U.S. states, MacKenzie and Goodstein (1985) examined differences on a number of prison adjustment variables. In contrast to offenders who were at an early point in their sentence (average time served 1.3 years), those subjects who had been imprisoned an average of 10.3 years reported less anxiety and fear of other inmates, less depression, fewer psychosomatic complaints, and higher self-esteem.

In summary, the available evidence indicates that gross psychological deterioration is not an inevitable consequence of imprisonment. However, the research may be criticized for using measures that are insensitive to subtle effects of imprisonment (Cohen and Taylor, 1972; Flanagan, 1982). In addition, the samples of prisoners that have been studied often have been nonrepresentative (e.g., they were selected after systematic attribution by parole release), and the effects of other potentially significant factors (e.g., age, prior prison experience) typically have not been adequately controlled for or taken into account. Finally, there is again the reliance on cross-sectional designs. Nevertheless, it cannot be denied that the psychological evidence to date is inconsistent with the view that imprisonment is generally or uniformly damaging.

From our perspective, this is not at all surprising. Conceptually, it makes little sense to search for the psychological effects of imprisonment without acknowledging that these effects may vary considerably across individuals. How individuals cope with problems is more important than the frequency or severity of problems they experience. Unfortunately, as with the sociological literature on imprisonment, previous psychological studies have concentrated on finding generalized and uniform effects. The reasons for variations among prisoners in social functioning and emotional or mental health have been typically ignored.

Other Consequences of Imprisonment

The implicit assumption that it is unimportant to deal with individual differences has also characterized other research related to the effects of imprisonment. Although we will consider it only briefly here, there is a fairly broad literature examining the effect of specific features of some prison environments, such as crowding and solitary confinement.

Among the many studies of the effects of prison crowding (Ellis, 1984; Gaes, 1985) little attention has been paid to the cognitive appraisal, coping, and attitudinal or personality variables that can moderate and mediate the experience of crowding (Bonta, 1986). This is the case in spite of the fact that the theoretical and experimental literature on crowding clearly points to the importance of person factors and their interaction with aspects of crowded environments (Stokols, 1972; Sundstrom, 1978).

The criminological literature on solitary confinement of inmates provides another example of assumed deleterious effects (Jackson, 1983). As in the previous cases, when we look at the research we find that there is no evidence for generalized negative effects, but there is again some evidence for beneficial effects, and there are clearly individual differences in response to such confinement (Gendreau and Bonta, 1984; Suedfeld, Ramirez, Deaton, and Baker-Brown, 1982).

Thus, our reading of the literature on the effects of particular features of the prison environment leads us to the same conclusion that we reached after surveying the larger bodies of work in the broader sociological and psychological areas. Once more, we see the need for consideration of the interaction between persons and environments.

Coping Theory

Finally, we come to the outline of our own theoretical perspective. Given the ideas in the section of this chapter on environmentalism versus nativism, and also the criticisms in our review of previous research on the effects of imprisonment, it should already be apparent that we wanted to focus on the interaction of personal and environmental factors. Since we were interested in predicting behavior that may be considered maladaptive, we thought it useful to adopt a conceptual framework that evolved from attempts to deal with the differences between adaptive and maladaptive responses to situations.

The conceptualization we chose was that of coping theory, especially as articulated by Lazarus and his associates (Lazarus, 1966, 1980; Lazarus, Averill, and Opton, 1970; Lazarus and Launier, 1978; Lazarus and Folkman, 1983). This set of constructs is a good expression of an attempt to operationalize the message of interactionism, and it is an excellent and well-articulated set of ideas for the study of the coping (adaptive) process.

An an example of how a description of coping behaviors can represent the interaction between the person and the objective reality of circumstances, consider two individuals who are facing a long prison sentence. Both experience the same environment, with the restrictions and deprivations that we will consider in more detail later. Given the objective reality, both will find that events that occur in prison are often beyond their control.

However, as a result of his individual history and attributes, e.g., acquired beliefs, reinforcement history, and innate capacities, one person will interpret the lack of control as the result of his own inadequacy. In contrast, the second individual interprets the situation as one where others have used and abused him and are continuing to do so. It is likely that the first person will sink into depression, apathy, and withdrawal; the second is more likely to become resentful, angry, and rebellious in an attempt to counter the control by others, even if it exacerbates his situation.

Similarly, the way that the same individuals actually deal with their long sentences will also determine how they are affected by the environment. Suppose that one individual deals with the stress of the long confinement he faces by avoiding all thoughts of the future, while the other strives to ameliorate his condition by finding a safe and comfortable behavioral niche within the institution.

The first person will likely immerse himself in the immate social network and take on the behavior and values of other prisoners; he will often be seen by outsiders as acting impulsively and carelessly. The second inmate will probably seem more rational and controlled to the outsider, with much weaker ties to the inmate subculture. These behaviors will in turn affect the ways the two men are seen by both staff and other prisoners, and their subsequent treatment will differ. All of this will also affect emotional responses and the ways our two individuals appraise their environments. And, of course, subsequent behavior will then be affected by each factor, continuously and continually.

Let us consider more generally how we can represent what happens when one copes with a problem situation. Lazarus argues that there are several steps occurring in the course of the coping process. First, there must be some potentially difficult situation, one that threatens the physical or psychologial safety or well-being of the individual. When such a situation occurs, it will present a demand for the person's attention.

However, cues from a potential problem situation alone do not constitute a threat. Rather, they must first be evaluated or appraised in terms of their significance to some aspect of the person's well-being. This first stage in the coping process has been labeled *primary appraisal*. The process of primary appraisal can result in the person's acknowledging and responding to a problem situation; alternatively, the individual may appraise the situation as harmless or irrelevant to himself, thus eliminating the need for further action. Thus, a situation must be appraised as threatening before it will evoke coping behavior, and the intensity of the perceived threat will probably also influence subsequent responding.

Having appraised an event or situation as threatening, the individual must also consider his alternatives for action. This is the second stage in the coping process. Lazarus uses the term *secondary appraisal* to refer to this evaluation of one's resources and options for responding. The results of the secondary appraisal are arrayed psychologically against the primary appraisal of the degree of threat in the situation, and from the comparison the person can decide how great a problem the situation really presents and whether he can master it to his satisfaction.

I should be noted that the terms *primary* and *secondary appraisal* are not intended to denote relative importance or even temporal ordering. Rather, the division emphasizes the different aspects of the appraisal task. The two parts of the appraisal process are clearly seen as influencing each other. The result of the judgment in primary appraisal will of course determine the (secondary) appraisal of what sort of actions are appropriate, while secondary appraisal can either mitigate or enhance the sense of threat that results from recognition of a problem in primary appraisal. In this regard, Lazarus has recognized that there may be some feedback among the elements of the appraisal process, with some reappraisal possible. This sort of mutual influence is characteristic of most accounts of complex cognitive processes, (Bandura, 1978), and it occurs at other stages of the coping process as well as during appraisal.

After appraisal, we would expect the person to respond to the threatening situation in some way. Of course, the actual response must be chosen from the set of possibilities that is available to the person, but the choice depends on the relative strength of each response within the person's repertoire, as well as the results of the appraisal process.

For example, if the situation is appraised as physically threatening, then the likely response will be one that the person has available to deal with such dangers. If in the past he has learned both to fight and to flee, then the choice in the current situation might be hard to predict, unless one knows which of the two he has done more commonly or more recently in similar situations. However, it is commonly assumed (without much real evidence) that most of us have relatively restricted repertoires for given types of situations, i.e., that we have characteristic "strategies" for coping with the types of problems we encounter, so prediction may often be fairly accurate.

There are, of course, a number of other important questions in the prediction of coping responses. Among them is the critical issue of how an individual acquires his repertoire of possible actions. For example, if one responds to a perceived threat by violent physical action, is this because he was reinforced for such behavior in the past, because he has seen others do so, or because he has some innate propensity for violence? Unfortunately, we do not know the answer to this question.

(As a result, it must be admitted that when we invoke "coping" to combine the working of both internal and external determinants of behavior we are not really solving the question of the acquisition of behavior, but only moving it back a level. However, the construct does allow us to represent the interaction of personal and situational variables on an everyday level; since this is the level of the events that we want to deal with, the construct is still important and useful even if it does not ultimately resolve the problem of the origin of behaviors in an individual.)

In any case, once a coping response has occurred, it completes the cycle in the theoretical set of events. However, the process does not stop there, for the act that occurs is only a single link in the continuous determinative chain of behavior. It is likely that almost any response will change the situation in which it occurs. Whether the change is major or trivial, it presents the person with a new situation to cope with and thus initiates a repetition of the appraisal and response processes. Thus, coping is really a continuous process; if we sometimes discuss particular responses by themselves, it is not because we believe that they occur in isolation, but rather that we find it easier to consider them one at a time.

As we shall consider in chapter 5, the resultant coping behaviors can be categorized and evaluated in a variety of ways. For example, if we maintain that the coping process has the purpose of alleviating problems or threats, then we can evaluate how well this is accomplished. There are a wide variety of ways that we can represent and discuss coping behavior, and we will employ several in the analyses reported in the following chapters.

This description focuses on the role of specific coping behaviors in response to particular problems, which may be either episodic or chronic. In addition, we can say that many of the more general ways we use to approach our environment are closely related to the elements of the coping process that we have described. For example, the extent to which we organize and plan our lives will influence the kinds of specific coping resources that we have available when we are faced with a problem; similarly, the specific things that we choose to do with our time, i.e., lifestyles, will determine the problems we encounter and how we can deal with them.

Thus, the study described in this monograph emphasized the central role of coping in the adaptive behavior of prison inmates, but it measured a wide variety of behaviors. The specifics of the methodology are presented in the next chapter, and most of the rest of this book will describe the results.

2
The Study: Design, Methods, Materials

Aims: What This Study Tried to Accomplish

With the perspective described above, we set out to study how prison inmates cope with their environment. To do this we needed to know what situations prisoners see as problems, how they interpret those problems, and, especially, what they do when they have a problem. The investigation of these questions was the core of our study.

In addition, we wanted to provide some data on more general aspects of offenders' behavior. We needed to know their personal histories and backgrounds, in order to relate these factors to their ways of coping. We also wanted to obtain a general picture of their more recent behavior and lifestyles on the outside, since we expected that general behavior patterns would interact with specific coping responses to affect outcomes. For example, difficulties in dealing with people may be less important for someone who leads a solitary lifestyle than for another person who spends a great deal of time socializing.

We were particularly interested in the effects of imprisonment and the way that confinement changes—or fails to change—established behavior patterns. Therefore, we decided to provide parallel sets of information about behavior outside and inside of prison. Thus, for example, we collected data on how inmates use their time while imprisoned and also similar data for their lives on the outside. Similarly, we compared individuals' coping under confinement with their coping with problems in the outside world. This parallelism was a distinctive feature of our study, and it will allow us to make a variety of interesting comparisons.

Of course, we were not restricted to studying only overt behavior. Although we approached the study of behavior from the coping-interactionist perspective described in chapter 1, it was important for us to look at a variety of different aspects of our subjects' lives. Looking at external behavior alone can lead one to a very parochial picture of people's lives, and in particular it can give a very distorted picture of offenders' lives. Therefore, we tried to gain some access to subjects' thoughts about how the world worked and their own places in it.

We did not seriously expect that we could ever gain access to our subjects' most private thoughts. In general, people are not themselves always aware of their most intimate thoughts and motives; if they are aware, it is sometimes difficult or impossible to articulate the material to another person; moreover, it is difficult to put such things into any standard form. Nevertheless, we did make some attempt to assess the role of cognitions in order to gain a more complete picture of inmates' behavior. Given our insistence on providing quantifiable data whenever possible, this involved mostly the use of standardized psychological tests to measure some aspects of cognitions which have been shown elsewhere to be important, although we added some scales of our own and also individual questions to delineate subjects' thoughts in particular situations. Thus, we made some effort to gather data on aspects of cognition which might be meaningfully measured, although we emphasized overt behavior.

Design Overview

The design of any investigation is critically important in determining the value of the results. With the particular difficulties of research in prisons, design considerations are even more complicated than they usually are. We expected that the effects of a prison term would develop over the course of time. Therefore, in studying how imprisonment affects people one must include some way of comparing across time. There are two basic ways of doing this: cross-sectional and longitudinal designs. In a cross-sectional study one compares groups of inmates who have already served different periods of time at the start of the investigation; in a longitudinal study one chooses a single group of subjects and follows them over time.

Most previous studies in the literature have used cross-sectional designs because they are far easier to execute in a prison setting. Access to prisoners is always restricted and often very difficult. If one needs to see the same individuals on several occasions, access at the required times is impossible to ensure. Even more, subjects may be permanently lost in a longitudinal design: some prisoners are released after a while, others are transferred a distance away, and still others are lost for a variety of reasons, from escape to refusal to cooperate any further with investigators. Also, if subjects are recruited in a single group, one can encounter an effect called cohort bias: some changes that reflect special characteristics of the sample or the time at which measurements are made may be visible, and these may be falsely interpreted as general effects of the situation.

On the other hand, there are even more serious problems with investigations using the cross-sectional method. Since they use different individuals to measure the effects of different lengths of imprisonment, one must match on any variables which may mediate the effects studied or which may affect the measures used, e.g., institutional conditions, age, prior prison experience, and many others. The difficulties become compounded when one considers that the factors one wants to control are often the basis of differential treatment across inmates. For example, age and prior prison experience are important considerations in everything from the choice of initial institutional assignment to the chances for early release.

In practice, satisfactory matching in cross-sectional designs is usually next to impossible. As a result, interpretation of the results is often problematic. One never knows whether any difference that appears between groups shows a real effect of the length of time in prison, or whether it is instead the result of one of the other extraneous variables. For example, one may end up comparing a mixed group of inmates who are beginning their terms with another group who have served several years. Any differences that appear might be the result of several years imprisonment, or they could be a selection artifact, since the latter group will undoubtedly consist of inmates who have been denied parole and are different from other inmates who were released on parole. Imperfect attempts at impossible requirements can often lead to confounded lies.

Thus, we saw ourselves faced with a choice between two difficult alternatives. At the end, our choice was clear, for several reasons. Even if proper matching could be achieved within a cross-sectional design, the results can be challenged. In order to measure the effects of time by comparing separate groups on a single occasion, one must assume that change occurs in a linear fashion across time and that individuals have changed at the same rate and to the same extent. These assumptions are probably incorrect, for people usually vary in the amount that they are affected by a given set of conditions or in the rate at which they change. Some prisoners may experience a strong distress syndrome early in their term, but gradually learn to adjust. Others may show an initial lack of reaction, with gradually increasing distress as they start to face the reality of their situations; still others may fall into cycles of distress and adaptation.

Since the cross-sectional method uses different subjects for each group, these individual differences cannot be seen easily. To look at coping and adaptation as we have conceived them, we need to follow the changes over time within individuals. Thus, we concluded that for our purposes the difficulties of a longitudinal design are in its execution, but the difficulties of a cross-sectional study are probably inherent in its logic, or at least in the fact that its assumptions are incompatible with common sense expectations about the ways that individuals adapt to the conditions they face.

There were also some features of a longitudinal method that were attractive for us. In addition to surveying the effects of the passage of time on behavior, we wanted to see if we could predict the course of adaptation. As we have conceived it, coping behaviors are ways of dealing with problem situations in order to resolve or remediate them. The success of current coping responses should be reflected in the quality of adaptation in the future. If we can meaningfully and reliably measure the quality of coping, then those measures should be capable of predicting adaptation in the future (as we have tried to do in chapter 10). In order to test such ideas, we needed to measure coping on one occasion and relate it to measures of subsequent adaptation.

Thus, we required the features of a longitudinal design to look at prediction of future behavior in addition to measuring current behavior. We attempted to avoid cohort effects by including subjects from a variety of settings and by recruiting them over a period of more than a year, so that any effects we saw could not be attributed to local or temporary conditions. We included several occasions for repeated measurements with each subject over a period of 16 months. This allowed us to look at changes over time in some particular behaviors, such as coping; it provided for a measure of the possible effects of imprisonment which was methodologically better than those used previously; and it allowed us to include elements of the prediction of behavior from one occasion to the next.

While all of these followed from our original objectives, they also made this study unique. Our emphasis on coping and on the interaction between the individual and his environment was of course a relatively new departure in itself, but it also led us to compare inmates' behavior on the outside with that in prison, within a longitudinal study of the effects of imprisonment starting near the beginning of a term. To our knowledge, there are no other studies in the literature that provide such information. (There are, of course, other longitudinal studies on similar issues. For reviews, and for more discussion of the virtues and problems of the design, see Farrington, Ohlin, and Wilson, 1986, or Farrington, 1979.)

Our aims and objectives led us to the choice of the basic design of the study, for the reasons described above. They also dictated many of the details of the research. Our principal goal was to describe and classify coping responses, but this had not been done before in any systematic fashion, and we were not sure what form the answers would take. Therefore, we devised a set of interview questions to elicit the desired information. We also wanted a variety of additional information to relate to the data on coping, and for this we included other questions in the interview, and also used previously established questionnaires in many cases. Finally, we needed data on how well our subjects adjusted and functioned in the prison environment, so we employed some institutional file measures.

We considered it important to not include anyone who would be unable to complete the requirements of the study, but at the same time we did not want to exclude too many inmates, lest the results become unrepresentative of the general prison population. As will be described below, this was accomplished reasonably well.

Once criteria for subjects were established, and the support and cooperation of the system had been arranged, we selected potential subjects and approached them to ask for their cooperation. When they agreed, they were interviewed and administered our set of questionnaires as soon as could be arranged. In order to assess changes, they were tested again after an interval of 3–4 months, and finally on a third occasion after an interval of about a year. After we had seen them for the last time, we obtained whatever file information was available.

With the abolition of the death penalty in Canada in 1976, mandatory life sentences had been established for a number of offenses, particularly first- and second-degree murder. In addition, (long) minimum terms had been mandated before offenders in these categories could be eligible to apply for parole. These minimum terms were especially severe for persons convicted of first-degree murder, who must now serve 25 years before they can be considered for parole. It was expected that the changes would lead to a very substantial increase in the number of long-term prisoners in the system, and for this reason we were particularly interested in the behavior and adjustment of men facing and serving these long sentences. Our selection of subjects aimed to ensure a high representation of inmates with long terms while still allowing our sample to yield representative figures for the entire population. We did this by grouping potential subjects according to the lengths of their sentences, and then selecting randomly within each group.

Details of the selection of subjects and the measures we used are in the following sections.

Setting

This study was conducted in the penitentiaries of the Ontario region of the Corrections Service of Canada. In this country, the responsibility for criminal law is primarily federal, and there is a uniform national criminal code. However, the responsibility for convicted offenders is arbitrarily divided between federal and provincial administration, so that anyone given a sentence by the court of 2 years or more is assigned to a federal penitentiary, while those with shorter sentences go to provincial prisons. Thus, we were dealing with offenders convicted of relatively serious crimes.

The Canadian federal system is divided into five regions for administrative purposes. The Ontario region is the largest, and it is fairly representative of the system as a whole. It contains about 30% of the entire federal prison population, which was just over 10,000 when we began this study and is now close to 12,000.

Within the region, there are a variety of institutions, and they can be ordered in terms of the levels of confinement which they provide. Both Kingston Penitentiary and Millhaven Institution are classified as maximum-security, with well-guarded perimeters and restricted movement within. Collins Bay, Joyceville, and Warkworth institutions are all classified as medium-security; their perimeter security is strict, but inmates have some freedom of movement within their walls, at least at designated times. There are also several minimum security prisons, including two farm institutions, which hold inmates who are judged to present no danger to the community. Each of these prisons had its own atmosphere and each presented different rules and physical conditions.

At the top of the security classification, Millhaven was clearly the "big house." Security was strict and necessarily so, with many of the country's most serious criminals confined within, although, as will be considered later, the majority of inmates confined there presented little danger under confinement and might have been assigned to some other institution. "The Haven" is the newest of the Ontario penitentiaries, built low and spread out, with uniform concrete blocks, and with closely monitored electronically operated doors controlling access to every corridor.

In contrast, Kingston Pen was physically the most imposing of all: built in 1835, its high limestone walls, dark passageways, and cells with high small windows reminded one of its connection to the medieval dungeon. The oldest, and formerly the most notorious prison in Canada, it had been replaced in its principal function by Millhaven after it was severely damaged in a riot in 1973. Aside from its use as a reception center when we began our study, it housed mostly inmates in protective custody.

There were also differences in the physical environments presented by the three medium-security institutions, but more important were the differences in the inmate populations created by deliberate assignment policies. Collins Bay contained (barely) a high proportion of young but experienced criminals, and gave us an impression of vigorous activity and constant movement in the central areas. In contrast, Joyceville was relatively sedate, with an older population and a less centralized design. Offenders who were thought to have the best chance of rehabilitation were sent to Warkworth, where the security level was a notch lower. Here, the buildings were lower and the perimeter was maintained by wire fences rather than walls, so one could walk between buildings and have some feeling of open space.

Given the differences in the reputations of these various institutions, one might expect some differences in inmates' behavior within them, particularly adjustment. When we selected potential subjects we did not consider institutional assignments, but we did have a sampling of subjects in each of the maximum- and medium-security prisons. In chapter 9 we will report some comparisons among them.

Since none of our subjects were initially sent to minimum-security institutions, we will be unable to include them in the comparisons. However, by the end of the study some subjects had been transferred to minimum-security institutions. Although too few were assigned to any single institution to warrant specific descriptions, these institutions generally provide more open living conditions, e.g., they have rooms instead of cells, and security is fairly unobtrusive. Any inmate determined to escape can rather easily accomplish it in a minimum-security institution, and almost all of the escapes in the system occur there.

In general, the Canadian federal system could be characterized as relatively humane. As the result of a series of parliamentary and other inquiries, the federal government had committed itself a few years previously to a policy of modernization of facilities and liberalization of conditions.

Although there were areas where the aims had not been accomplished, some real progress had been made. At the time of the study, crowding was not a problem (although it is now) and every inmate had a cell of his own, about 6' by 9', with toilet and cold-water washing facilities contained; hot water was available in some cells, and the goal was to bring it to the rest. Under ordinary custody, inmates were allowed to be out of their cells about half of the time, for work or school and some recreation. Each institution had a variety of work placements and training facilities. Inmates were allowed open access to legal consultation, mail was not censored under ordinary circumstances, and conditions were monitored by citizens' advisory committees, although there was some criticism of the committees' effectiveness. There was also an ombudsman's office within the system, along with a set of procedures that inmates could use to appeal decisions with which they disagreed.

To be sure, for most of us these conditions would be quite unpleasant, and in many cases they were worse than described above. For example, although Kingston Pen had plumbing in each cell, it served as easy access conduits for the colonies of mice and rats which infested the building. Training programs were available, but the choices were always very limited, and sometimes there was a waiting list of up to a year for assignment to a preferred program. For many inmates, the bureaucracy was often inscrutable and impenetrable when they wanted changes in their situation. Still, as prisons go, the existing conditions were relatively favorable, the result of over a decade of effort to humanize the system. Ir addition, there was pressure for further change, as part of a widespread movement to broaden the recognized legal rights of Canadian citizens. However, there was also some backlash among the general public, with feelings that prisoners were treated rather too well, much of it fed by the inaccuracies and omissions of mass media reporting.

At the time this study was begun, convicted offenders were first sent to Kingston Penitentiary, where they were assessed for assignment to one of the other federal institutions in the region. In practice, it was very rare for an inmate to be assigned initially to minimum security. When we had tested about half of our initial complement of subjects the Reception Centre was closed, and subsequently inmates were assigned to a receiving institution shortly after sentencing. Since the initial assignment of inmates was quite conservative under both systems, the change appeared to have little effect, and later analyses could find no differences between inmates assigned under the two methods (although there were probably some effects across the system that became visible later, as discussed in the 1984 Carson commission report (Communications Division, 1984)).

Finally, we should note that conditions in the Ontario penitentiary system were relatively stable during the time we were gathering data. Shortly after we finished, the number of inmates in the system rose significantly, and crowding became a problem. At about the same time (although not necessarily related), a rash of violent incidents began, including murders and suicides. Fortunately, our data preceded this period of unrest, so they reflect what happens in a period of relative calm. Unfortunately, we can say very little about what happens during times of disturbance.

Measures and Materials

To get the broad picture of lifestyle, coping, and cognitions that we wanted, we needed to use a variety of sources of data. The most important was a highly structured interview which we devised for the purpose. This gathered a great deal of information on actual behaviors, directly from the subject. However, we also asked our subjects to complete a variety of standardized questionnaires. Most of these were selected to measure particular emotional states and/or cognitions, e.g., depression or the attribution of control; the versions we used had generally been used before with some success in the psychological literature. We also devised a few questionnaires of our own when we could find no good published instruments to measure certain things. The final source of data was institutional files, which were usable for some confirmation of background information and also for some data on behavior during the prison term, such as disciplinary and medical problems.

The various data-gathering instruments had been tested and revised several times during preliminary stages of the study, the details of which were reported in an interim contract report for the Ministry of the Solicitor General (Zamble and Porporino 1980), and summarized in the final contract report (Zamble, Porporino, and Kalotay, 1984). The purpose of the preliminary work had been to ensure the ease and practicality of administering the various measures, and especially to check that questions were clear to inmates and yielded clear answers. Trial versions of the interview and the questionnaires we originated were administered to small samples of inmates for feedback and revision. In the final preliminary stage we subjected our interview protocol to a test of interrater reliability, with modification or deletion of items that did not provide reliable information.

Following are some details of the final versions of each of our sources of data.

THE STRUCTURED INTERVIEW

The initial interview contained three basic sections, each with a focus on information from a different aspect of the respondent's life. The complete protocol is included in the Appendix. The first section covered background and historical measures, including family, education, employment, criminal history, and a variety of other aspects of personal history. There were also questions about current circumstances, such as the current offense and sentence, and also expectations regarding the current term of imprisonment.

This section of the interview was intended to function as an easy-flowing introduction, with straightforward questions to which there were were mostly factual answers, in order to establish some rapport between the inmate and the interviewer. At the same time, some of the questions, e.g., one regarding previous suicide attempts, were intended to give an early indication that questions of a relatively probing and intimate nature would be an integral part of the interview.

In the second section of the interview we asked subjects to tell about their behavior on the outside, before they had been charged with their current offenses. The emphasis was on a survey of the problems they had encountered and on the ways they had dealt with those problems, but there were a variety of other questions to allow us to form a picture of their lifestyles on the outside. For example, we asked what they had done with their time, how they had organized their days, and how often they had thought of their past and future.

We wanted to avoid leading our subjects into answering in ways that would have fit our prior expectations, but at the same time we wanted definite answers to our questions and we wanted those answers to allow easy quantification or classification. Therefore, in many cases we adopted a strategy of inquiry that might be called *progressive focusing*. We would begin with an entirely open-ended question, allowing the subject to give his immediate and unconstrained response. In most cases we found that such inquiries elicited little information, which is understandable when we consider that subjects were unlikely to be currently thinking about most of the areas we were interested in. The relevant information had to be recalled from memory. Therefore, we followed the initial inquiry with other questions that were progressively more specific, until we had asked about all aspects of the original question, even if the subject had not originally volunteered them. We hoped that this technique would help the subject to recall comprehensive information on various aspects of his life without forcing his answers in any direction.

This method of focusing was used most prominently in finding the problems which the subject had perceived in his life. We began by asking, "What problems were you experiencing?" Usually, this brought us only fragmentary information, so we then asked about broad classes of problems ("Did you have any problems at work?"), expecting that this would provide cues for the subject to search his memory and elicit more information. After the broad categories, we usually proceeded to a much more specific set of possible problems, eventually covering a variety of areas.

Thus, even if a subject could originally recall very little about his problems, we usually ended with a fairly comprehensive list. It was still possible that a subject had specified some problems only because of our suggestions, so at the end we reviewed all of the items on the list. We asked whether each had really been a problem, and had the subject arrange the final set of problems in the order of perceived importance.

The ordered list of problems was then used for the next major area of the interview, the examination of how the subject coped with his problems. For this purpose, we chose three problems from the subject's list. Usually, they were the three which were ranked highest, but sometimes the problems at the top of the list were very similar, so we chose one which was ranked lower. In a few cases, there were less than three problems on the final list.

For each of the problems chosen, we asked an extensive series of questions, again progressively more specific, to find out as much as we could about how the subject had dealt with the situation. We attempted to elicit a complete description of all types of behavior used, adaptive or maladaptive, immediate or delayed, spontaneous or planned, repeated or episodic.

The interview contained a variety of specific questions based on Lazarus's typology of coping responses categorized according to their purpose or function (e.g., Lazarus and Launier, 1978). However, we found that subjects did not respond to our questions as we had expected, for their answers did not correspond to the categories of the questions. That is, if we asked a question about attempts to find a solution for a given problem we might get an answer that told how the problem was avoided; if we asked about avoidance we might hear about attempts at emotional palliation, etc. In general, respondents seemed to act as though the different inquiries were merely repetitions of the same basic question, "What did you do?" We concluded that people do not categorize their coping responses according to their purpose, but rather as a loosely organized set of actions tied to the problem or situation which evokes them. Still, we found it useful to retain most of the sequence of questions, because the repetition often elicited a rich and varied set of replies, and we wanted as full a set of responses as possible.

In addition to the questions about problems and coping, we also asked about several other aspects of behavior and lifestyle. We attempted to cover the use of time, relationships with other people, and specific behaviors that may be useful in coping, e.g., daydreaming.

A final set of questions in the section about life on the outside dealt with the possible relationship between inmates' criminal offenses and the problems they were experiencing. We tried to find whether they saw any possible links with either their particular problems or the way they had dealt with problems.

After the extensive questioning about about life on the outside, the final part of the interview was concerned with life in prison. The questions were similar to those in the second section, with parallel questions wherever possible, so as to facilitate comparisons of behavior in prison with that in the outside world.

As in the second section, there was a concentration on problems and coping. Since the environment in prison is somewhat more predictable and less varied than that on the outside, we were able to be more specific in the listing of likely difficulties. We were guided in part by Toch's (1977) classification of sources of stress in prison, but we also relied heavily on our own clinical experience in the setting. The sequence for eliciting a set of coping behaviors was identical to that used with problems outside of prison. Other questions in this section were mostly like those in the preceding section, except that there were some items about situations unique to prison, e.g., spending time in one's cell.

The entire interview usually took about 1 1/2 hours, normally in a single sitting. Although it is difficult to become physically comfortable in a sparsely furnished interview room, we worked to put subjects at ease and to establish some trust. Most of the interviews were conducted by a mature female research assistant, while the others were done by the first author. Both attempted to be sympathetic to the concerns of the inmates, and cooperation was generally excellent.

This was possible because we were identified as outsiders, and because we promised—and maintained—confidentiality. We worked carefully to establish a position of trust, and we believe that we were successful. After the first few interviews in each institution, information about us had reached the local rumor networks, and some inmates agreed to participate as soon as we introduced ourselves, even before we had given our customary explanations about the investigation.

Sometimes inmates claimed to be telling us things that they had never discussed with anyone before. While this was probably an exaggeration at times, we were heartened by the fact that subjects very rarely refused to answer any question. Often they told us things that would have been very damaging to their reputations, either in prison or on the outside, e.g., how they had cheated their inmate friends or committed crimes for which they had not been charged. Many of them were obviously lonely, and wanted someone to talk with, and the presence of a neutral outsider was uncommon within the institutions, so our most common problem was to complete the interviews within reasonable time limits.

Occasionally, a subject began to tell us about future misbehavior, such as planned escape attempts. We were bound to report such information, but to do so would have compromised our neutrality, so we cut them off before we heard too much, despite our curiosity. In a few other cases we felt we were being misled, and we then confronted the inmate with our disbelief; this usually produced some corrections or clarification. A few times we disbelieved the stories we were given, and decided to check them when the subject maintained that they were true. When we looked at the information that was available in official files, we decided that the inmate had probably told us the truth.

We believe that most subjects were open and honest with us, and that the information they gave us was accurate, at least to the extent of their awareness. Although verification of this opinion is impossible, there would have been little reason for inmates to give false information, especially when the information we wanted had very little to do with their criminal cases. We concluded that in general our interview reports were at least as accurate as other sources of data.

We were able to make direct comparisons on some measures, for example histories of prior criminal convictions and imprisonment. In these categories, information obtained in our interviews was identical with that in files for 85–90% of our cases. Where there was disagreement, some checking indicated that the interview data were probably at least as accurate as files. In the great majority of cases of disagreement the interview data included reports of offenses or sentences that were not listed in official files. When we checked with subjects, we learned that files had omitted items for a variety of reasons, e.g., offenses had been committed under false names or in another country, and were not known to the authorities, although subjects included them in their accounts during the interview.

QUESTIONNAIRE MEASURES

In addition to the interview, we also used a set of questionnaires. These were given to subjects after they had completed the interview, usually in a separate session. Where it was possible, we administered the questionnaires to groups of 2–5 inmates, but we were careful to check this in advance with each subject. Sometimes a subject had some worries about his reading ability and wanted help with the questionnaires, and in these cases we saw them individually. Sometimes there were other reasons why subjects had to be seen individually, such as the conditions of their confinement.

Questionnaires were chosen primarily as measures of emotional and cognitive states. For the assessment of emotional adjustment we tried to choose scales which had both good clinical relevance and also well-established reliability. Measures of cognitive states were used if they had been previously shown to have some relevance to the behavior of prisoners. While most of the scales we used had had extensive previous use, in a few cases we were unable to find anything that met our requirements, so we devised some new ones.

Among reactions to stressful events, anxiety and depression are central. Certainly, the literature on the psychological consequences of imprisonment makes recurring references to the pervasiveness of anxiety and depression among inmates. The state anxiety (A-state) scale of the Stait–Trait Anxiety Inventory (STAI; Spielberger, Gorsuch, and Lushene, 1970) was chosen to assess levels of current anxiety. This scale is quite brief and it is well accepted in the literature as a measure of anxiety state (Smith and Lay, 1974).

As a primary measure of depression we chose the Beck Depression Inventory (BDI; Beck, 1967). It is relatively short and widely used for the assessment of depressive symptomatology. In addition, we used the Beck Hopelessness Scale (Beck, Weissman, Lester, and Trexler, 1974) as a measure of enduring depression. Depressive mood can be a common reaction to any major negative event in life, such as the beginning of a term in prison, but one would usually expect it to be transitory. However, hopelessness is probably characteristic of more enduring depression, and it has been shown to be a measure of suicidal ideation (Beck, Kovacs, and Weissman, 1979). Finally, to serve as an ancillary measure of mood state and change, we used a brief adjective checklist, using 42 items from the Multiple Adjective Check List (Zuckerman and Lubin, 1965) and the Profile of Mood States (McNair, Lorr, and Droppleman, 1971).

Self-esteem is usually considered to be an important determinant of general emotional state and one of the principal cognitive mediators of behavior. Some previous studies have looked at the impact of imprisonment on self-esteem but the results are inconsistent (Bennett, 1974; Gendreau, Grant, and Leipciger, 1979; Hepburn and Stratton, 1977; Reckless and Dinitz, 1970). We expected that much of the confusion might be attributable to differences in the time of measurement or from an interaction with coping, so we included a measure of this construct, a brief 20-item scale made of 10 items from the Coopersmith Self-Esteem Inventory (Coopersmith, 1967) and 10 items from the self-depreciation scale of the Basic Personality Inventory (Jackson, 1976).

Another major cognitive construct which we expected to affect behavior in prison was locus of control (Rotter, 1966). This is a measure of the tendency of individuals to make generalized attributions about the causation of events, particularly whether (and how much) they see events in their lives as controlled by external forces rather than by their own actions. There have been studies of the relationship between locus of control measures and coping (Anderson, 1977); it has also been noted that perceived loss of personal control could be expected to be a basic response to imprisonment (McKay, Jayewardene, and Reedie, 1977). We used two scales to measure this construct. The first was a version of Rotter's Internal-External scale (Rotter, 1966).

In addition, we constructed a scale to be specifically relevant to the experience of imprisonment. The Prison Control Scale is made up of 40 items designed to cover a variety of events in prison life, e.g., getting a work change, respect by other inmates, etc. As in other locus of control scales, respondents are asked to indicate how much control they think they have over each sort of event, and the scale is then scored for total perceived control. A preliminary testing conducted by Porporino (1983) showed a high internal consistency (coefficient alpha = .91). It was also found to differentiate significantly between inmates classified by case management staff as either coping well or coping badly. A copy of the complete scale is included in the Appendix, along with a summary of the reliability and item-analyses from Porporino (1983).

Criminal attitudes and belief systems have been consistently implicated in criminological theory and in research on the antecedents of criminal behavior. Styles of adaptation in prison have also been related to criminal attitudes (Irwin, 1970; Thomas and Petersen, 1977). The attitude measure we used in this study was one adapted from scales used in the Connecticut Correctional System (Gendreau and Gibson, 1970). This scale has been administered to large numbers of federal and provincial offenders in Ontario and its validity statistics are good (Andrews and Wormith, 1983). It has also been shown to be useful in measuring the effects of correctional treatment programs (Wormith, 1980).

As a measure of primary appraisals of problems in prison, we developed a 40-item inventory of common concerns of prisoners. The items in the Prison Problems Scale were based on those mentioned in the works of Toch (1975, 1977), and Cohen and Taylor (1981) but they included others from our clinical experience with inmates and from preliminary work on this study. Previous testing (Porporino, 1983) had indicated that this scale had high internal consistency (coefficient alpha = .93) and that it could differentiate between inmates seen by staff members as coping either well or poorly. A copy of the complete scale is included in the Appendix, along with a summary of the reliability and item-analyses from Porporino (1983).

The other scales used were chosen to measure additional items of particular interest. The first was intended to check for some possible biases in the measurement process. A problem with self-report scales is that respondents may attempt to present themselves in an unrealistically favorable light. This sort of distortion of answers, commonly called a social desirability response bias by psychometricians, might be particularly serious with a population of convicted criminal offenders. Therefore, we used a shortened version (Strahan and Gerbasi, 1972) of the Marlowe–Crowne Social Desirability Scale (Crowne and Marlowe, 1960), a scale that has been used extensively to detect "faking-good" responses.

After the data had been gathered, correlations were calculated between the Social Desirability scores and a wide variety of other measures. A table of all of the significant correlations with Social Desirability, as measured at the initial interview, is presented as an Appendix. Only a few of the set of correlations calculated reached statistical significance, and those that did were low. For only one variable did the relationship with Social Desirability account for even 10% of the variance: the results of this measure (the Self-Depreciation Scale) will be omitted from any further discussion. Otherwise, we concluded that the effects of social desirability did not play an important role in biasing subjects' reporting, and the results from this scale will not be discussed further.

However, it should be noted that the lack of a social desirability bias is not surprising: even if subjects were disposed toward biased responding, on most of our questions it would not have been clear what was a socially desirable answer. Nevertheless, it is reassuring to be able to show that our data were not largely influenced by subjects giving us answers they thought we might like to hear.

Another measure of interest was the occurrence of major events in subjects' lives in the period preceding their offenses. Research in the last decade has made it clear that there is a relationship between measures of the occurrence of major events in one's life and subsequent physical and emotional disturbances (Dohrenwend and Dohrenwend, 1973; Gunderson and Rahe, 1974; Moos, 1976). In light of this, we wondered about the relationship between stressful life events and criminal offenses. In considering the response to imprisonment, we also felt that the events in a person's life previous to imprisonment might affect how he reacts to imprisonment. We used the Life Experiences Survey (Sarason, Johnson, and Siegel, 1978), although we made a few modifications to include some common experiences of offenders, e.g., being pursued by police. We also devised a Prison Life Events Scale to be used at the final interview. This questionnaire listed a series of events that might happen during a term in prison, and it was scored similarly to the scales counting events on the outside.

The final scale included was an inventory of drug use on the outside in the period before imprisonment. Since the use of drugs is very common as a coping behavior, it was important for us to gather some quantitative information on usage, both as indications of the drug abuse problem in itself and to relate to other aspects of behavior. Our scale was derived from that of Lightfoot-Barbaree and Barbaree (1979) but with very extensive revisions.

It was necessary to limit the number of scales administered at each testing. We expected that fatigue would become a problem for subjects after an hour of filling out forms. Some subjects needed help with reading, and this extended considerably the time necessary for completion. Therefore, a different subset of scales was chosen to be given after each of the three interviews. The important emotional measures were administered all three times, but most other scales were given only once or twice. The schedule for administration of each scale is shown in Table 2.1, along with a summary of when other sources of data were gathered.

FILE MEASURES

The last category of data was gathered from institutional files. We had originally expected that file data could be used to validate much of the information we obtained from subjects, but this was not possible.

Since they were often very incomplete, files were even less reliable as sources of information on other aspects of inmates' personal histories. For example, information on basic family background or socioeconomic levels was missing in about half of the cases. In retrospect, this should not have

TABLE 2.1. Schedule for administration of measures.

Data source	Testing occasion		
	1	2	3
Interview			
Part A (background)	×		
Part B (life outside)	×		
Part C (life inside)	×	×	×
Questionnaires			
Spielberger State Anxiety Inventory	×	×	×
Beck Depression Inventory	×	×	×
Hopelessness Scale	×	×	×
Mood Adjective Checklist	×	×	×
Life Events Scale	×		
Prison Life Events Scale			×
Locus of Control Scale	×		×
Prison Locus of Control Scale		×	×
Self-Esteem and Self-Depreciation	×		×
Social Desirability Scale	×		×
Attitudes to Legal System Scale	×		×
Prison Problems Scale		×	×
Drug Use Inventory	×		
File Data			
Disciplinary			
Days lost privileges			×
Days in punitive dissociation			×
Days earned remission lost			×
Institutional job changes			×
Institutional transfers			×
Medical			
Initiations or requests for attention			×
Diagnoses and descriptions of complaints			×
Prescribed medications			×

been surprising, since files are kept by institutions to provide current and necessary information, and a person's childhood history is not particularly relevant to management of his current sentence. Moreover, background information that did appear in the files had usually been obtained from the inmate during interviews by institutional staff, so it was comparable in reliability to the data we obtained in our own interviews, except that our data were usually more complete.

In any case, we decided to make use of files only for information that we could not obtain from inmates themselves. In particular, this included files on disciplinary offenses, which were usually carefully documented and included information not always made available to inmates, and also medical treatment records, which often contained information that inmates might not know or understand, such as names of prescribed medications or final diagnoses of presenting conditions.

3
Subjects: Selection and Characteristics

Selection and Recruitment

Before recruiting subjects for the study, we set up a series of requirements. In the first place, we decided to deal only with male prisoners. There are roughly 100 men in federal institutions in Canada for every woman. Moreover, there are major differences between the ways that men and women are treated in prison, and probably in their ways of adaptation as well (cf., Heffernan, 1972), so we could not easily treat women as a subgroup within the male population. Thus, we realized that we could not study both men and women; for this study we considered the numbers and chose to deal only with male prisoners.

The selection of subjects began in October 1980, and continued until April 1982. Potential subjects were chosen from lists of new inmates that we obtained from the regional headquarters (Ontario) of the Correctional Service of Canada.

We wanted to have the initial interview take place as close to the beginning of the sentence as possible, so we excluded the occasional offender who had been sentenced more than about a month before being transferred to a federal institution. Because we had scheduled followup interviews over a period of 16 months, we required that potential subjects have a new term of at least two years, the usual minimum sentence for a federal institution. This criterion excluded offenders returning to serve the end of a sentence after parole revocation with no major new convictions.

After applying the above criteria, the choice of potential subjects was random with one constraint. In order to assess the effects of length of sentence, the sample was divided into short-term (less than 5 years), medium-term (5–10 years), and long-term (10 years to life) offenders. Although we wanted to end up with about the same number of subjects in each of these subgroups, they were not equally represented in the population of inmates admitted to federal institutions. Therefore, selection was conducted randomly—but separately—for each of the three subgroups, with the proportion sampled varying according to the number of new inmates in each group. Since there were far fewer new inmates in our long-term category than in the other two groups, we selected nearly all long-termers who arrived during the sampling period.

When the names of potential subjects had been selected, they were first submitted to a contact person in each institution, usually a psychologist. The names were screened to eliminate those who were unlikely to be able to meet the requirements of the study. Senior security officers in each institution were also asked to identify those who might present a threat to the safety of an interviewer. Of the 184 potential subjects whose names were submitted, a total of 17 were screened out in this process. Five individuals were eliminated because of inadequate command of English, 1 was judged to be totally illiterate, 5 others were either psychotic or too agitated to interview, 2 were mentally defective (including 1 with a recent head injury), and 4 were screened out by security staff.

The remaining potential subjects were scheduled individually for brief consent interviews in which we introduced ourselves, provided a written summary of the aims and procedures of the study, and answered questions. Each potential subject was assured that his responses would be treated with full confidentiality and that he had the option of withdrawing at any time. The inmate was then asked whether he was willing to participate. If he agreed to participate, he was asked to sign a consent form indicating his willingness to give the investigators access to his case management, security, and medical files. (Copies of the information and consent forms are included in the Appendix.) A total of 15 inmates declined to participate when asked; 4 others agreed but changed their minds before completion of the first interview and testing session.

For a variety of reasons, a third group of potential subjects was unavailable for either the consent interview or the data-gathering interview and testing. The reasons for their absence were almost always unique, and entirely unrelated to the study, e.g., temporarily transferred for trial, escaped from custody, etc. The majority of these actually had appeared at the consent interview and agreed to participate, but they were not available for interviews afterwards. A total of 15 inmates were lost in this category.

The various reasons for the loss of potential subjects are listed in Table 3.1. If one eliminates those who were not available, the potential subject pool consisted of 169 individuals. Of these, the 133 who participated consituted about 79%, including a refusal rate of about 11% and 10% who were eliminated in preliminary screening. There were 45 subjects in our short-term group, 47 in the medium-term, and 41 long-termers. There was some further attrition over the course of the study, with 130 completed second interview-testings and a drop to 98 interviews completed at the final (third) scheduled occasion. Almost all of the losses after the first interview were the result of subjects being released for various reasons; as might be expected, the loss were heaviest in the short-term group, many of whom were paroled.

TABLE 3.1. Disposition of potential subjects.

	Length of sentence			
	Short	Medium	Long	Total
Original sample	58	66	60	184
Losses				
Screened out	5	8	4	17
Refused	5	4	10	19
Unavailable	3	7	5	15
Included in study	45	47	41	133

Characteristics: Sentences, Offenses, Criminal History

This section summarizes some of the general characteristics of our sample. One question to consider is whether the individuals we studied were representative of the general population of Canadian penitentiary inmates. Therefore, Table 3.2 presents some summary characteristics of the sample along with values for the Canadian federal system as a whole at the time of sampling (Corrections Services in Canada, 1982).

Of course, we would expect that sentence length would be longer than average, given our method of blocking to include a high proportion of inmates with very long terms. In fact, the distortion was not that great, for about one-quarter of inmates admitted to federal penitentiaries during the time of the study had sentences of from 10 years to life, as opposed to slightly less than a third in our sample. In the other direction, our sample had a low proportion of inmates with sentences of between 2 and 5 years. This group comprised about 44% of the total population but only about one-third of the sample.

Most of the inmates in our sample had been imprisoned for principal current offenses which were serious and violent. The two most frequent offenses categories, with virtually identical numbers, were robbery and murder (including manslaughter). A total of 58% were serving sentences for violent crimes, which is within the range of 55–60% in the last decade for the Canadian federal system as a whole.

The sample can also be compared to general prison population figures in terms of age, and again it appears fairly representative. The ages at the first interview ranged from 17 to 63, with a mean age very close to the mean age of admission in 1980 for the system (Inform, 1985). About 10% were under 21, but the modal age group was from 21 to 30, which included about half of all subjects.

The men in this study also seemed typical of the federal prison population in their previous criminal history. Official summaries in the past decade have indicated that, as a rough rule of thumb, about one-third of men beginning federal terms have previously served such terms (2 years or

TABLE 3.2. Characteristics of subject sample and comparisons to overall CSC values.

Variable	Sample	Overall system
Sentence length[a]		
Mean (months)	115.0	—[b]
Percent		
24–59 months	34.0	44.0[c]
60–119 months	35.0	23.0[c]
120 months to life	30.0	26.0[c]
Mean age	29.8	27.9
Principal current offense		
Theft, burglary, other property	17.0	22.0
Drug offenses	13.0	10.0
Robbery	28.0	30.0
Assault or wounding	3.0	3.0
Sex offenses	4.0	8.0
Murder, manslaughter	27.0	19.0
Other	8.0	7.0
Previous imprisonment		
Percent with previous penitentiary	32.0	36.0
Mean terms (those with previous penitentiary)	1.7	—[b]
Percent with previous reformatory	68.0	—[b]
Means terms (those with previous reformatory)	2.9	—[b]
Percent with any previous prison	72.0	—[b]
Custody level (first interview)		
Maximum security	27.0	—[b]
Medium security	68.0	—[b]
Minimum security	0.0	—[b]
Protective custody	5.0	—[b]

[a] For life sentences, the value used in calculating mean sentence length is the minimum time until parole eligibility.
[b] Comparable figures not available.
[c] These percentages do not sum to 100 because of inmates who have been returned for violation of release terms (and who are classified according to time remaining when reimprisoned, often less than 2 years).

over), two-thirds have previously been in provincial institutions for terms of less than 2 years, and about one-third have never before been in prison. Our sample more or less followed this rule, with 32% who had been in a penitentiary (and probably also had been in provincial institutions), 68% who had been imprisoned in provincial institutions, and only 28% who had not been in prison. This split is fortuitous, as we will see later, for it allows us to make some interesting comparisons according to previous prison experience.

Thus, for the most part we were dealing with experienced criminals, and many had extensive histories of previous imprisonment. We calculated that the mean length of previous imprisonment for the entire sample was 47 months; considering the subset who had no previous terms, and the age of the sample, this is an impressive figure. Moreover, 20% had been sentenced to a correctional term before the age of 16, and over 40% before 18, even though courts had been generally loathe to imprison juveniles.

In summary, we can say that the pattern of criminal offenses shown by our subjects varied considerably. Often it was long and persistent, showing most of the characteristics of hard-core or career offenders, including a start at an early age and a high rate of offenses. On the other hand, some subjects had no recorded history of previous criminal acts. The total number of officially recorded convictions varied from 1—the current offense— to a high of 54, with a median of just over 11. Interestingly, inmates in the long-term group tended to have shorter records: about half of them had not been in prison before. Thus, the sample included a considerable diversity in terms of previous criminal offenses, from a group of habitual criminals to a group of men who seemed to have fallen into a single catastrophic act. In this diversity, the subjects in this study present a fair sample of the men in our penitentiaries.

Social and Economic Background

Having established that we are dealing with perpetrators of serious criminal acts, we might ask what factors in the histories of these men could have led to such behaviors. One of the more pervasive myths in our folklore about criminal behavior is the idea that offenders are typically the products of social and economic deprivation. However, from the interactionist standpoint we would expect that such conditions would be only one of a number of factors that might dispose a person toward criminal acts. Deprivation should have little in the way of direct causative effects, but rather it ought to act only in combination with other determinants. While there would be a statistical link between socioeconomic factors and criminality, the link should be weak. Most individuals who grow up even in the most deprived circumstances should be law-abiding and nonviolent, and conversely, many criminals would have no evidence of any deprivation in their background.

This is generally what we see in the social and economic histories of our subjects, as summarized in Table 3.3. For example, if we use the father's occupation as an index of economic status, we find that many of our subjects came from relatively poor families. Only 28% of their fathers had skilled, managerial, or executive occupations, while 45% worked in semiskilled or clerical positions, and the rest worked as laborers or in unskilled jobs. Compared to Canadian society as a whole, very heavily weighted in the middle-class categories, we could conclude that our sample was disadvantaged. Still, a wide range of economic origins was included. Although average economic class origins for subjects were probably lower than those for a randomly chosen sample of the nonimprisoned population, we found representations from all classes. At the extremes, while 3 sub-

TABLE 3.3. Social and family backgrounds of subjects.

Variable	
Racial background (%)	
Caucasian	87.8
Native American	6.5
Black	4.1
Asiatic or other	1.6
Citizenship (%)	
Native-born Canadian	87.2
Naturalized Canadian	8.8
Other	4.0
Father's occupation (%)	
Unskilled or none	27.3
Semi-skilled or sales	44.6
Skilled	24.0
Professional or managerial	4.1
Social class estimate (%)	
Poverty/lower class	32.7
Working class	38.9
Middle class or higher	28.3
Family size and birth order	
Mean total family size	3.4
Only-born (%)	7.5
Firstborn (including only-born) (%)	29.5
Percent with siblings who have prison records	
(excluding only-born)	32.2
Family intactness at ages 6–11 (%)	
Nuclear family intact	62.7
Nuclear family, one parent	18.6
Adoptive or extended family	8.5
Foster home or institution	10.2

jects had fathers who were chronically unemployed, the fathers of 5 others were practicing professionals.

A similar result is seen from our estimate of social class of the family of origin, estimated from information available in case management files. Only 28% of the families were classfied as clearly middle-class, with almost a third showing some evidence of economic deprivation. This latter figure is probably an overestimate, because for about half of the cases the files did not have enough information for us to form reasonable estimates of class origin, and we expect that the information would have more likely been recorded when poverty had been evident. Still, we can say that at least 1 in 6 subjects came from an impoverished background. Again, we see circumstances that seem disadvantaged when compared to the general population, but the difference is not so large as one might expect.

Despite common preconceptions, this is not surprising. Socioeconomic factors are rarely very powerfully related to criminality in contemporary

studies, especially those in Canadian populations. The strongest relationships were shown in English populations at the beginning of the century, where it was sometimes claimed that virtually all habitual offenders
came from the "lower" classes. However, in our society, class differences
are not nearly so profound, nor is a person's class affiliation fixed or uniformly defined. While social class still plays some role in modern English
investigations, such as the Cambridge longitudinal study (West and Farrington, 1973) it is weaker than in the older data. Among contemporary
Canadian studies, such as Offord's studies of delinquency among Ottawa
teenagers (Offord, 1982), the relationship becomes almost trivial, about
the level seen in our data.

Indices of most other aspects of social background show even less that
distinguishes our sample from a randomly chosen group of adult males in
Ontario. As can be seen in Table 3.3, almost all were Caucasian Euro-
peans; among other groups, only native Indians were overrepresented,
comprising 6% of the sample. Most of our subjects were also native-born
Canadian citizens.

Thus, just as the class influences seen in English studies are less important in a Canadian context, the racial and ethnic divisions which pervade
the American data are absent. This is not to say that Canadians do not
discriminate against minority groups to the same degree, given the chance.
However, until very recently Ontario society has always been characterized by a relative homogeneity. In addition, there is no extensive history of
official discrimination to match that in most other Western countries. Only
the non-European native groups have had a history of officially directed
discrimination, and they form only a small proportion of the population in
the region of this study.

Certainly, this does not mean that race and ethnicity played no part
in the criminal histories of our subjects. However, it was clearly a minor
factor in most cases, putting the lie to ideologies which see crime as the
product of class or ethnic conflicts, or as a way for one group to maintain
control over others. Although we can see little evidence for the direct influence of socioeconomic factors, crime is still a major problem in Canada,
so we look for explanations in other areas.

Although general socioeconomic conditions seem to show little that distinguishes offenders from the general population, we do have some evidence that the early environment is a determinant of criminal behavior.
Among the data shown in Table 3.3, some specific measures of family history and behavior show fairly sizable problems. For example, while 63% of
our subjects lived with intact nuclear families in their early school years—
between the ages of 6 and 11–19% were in broken nuclear families, 8%
lived with relatives other than parents, and 19% were in foster homes or
institutions. The last figure is several times the percentage of children
reared under governmental care in Ontario, and it shows clear evidence of
an unusual amount of family instability among our sample. This finding

replicates that of Offord (1982), which showed a strong link between family intactness and delinquency among Ottawa youth.

There was also evidence of problems within families during the early school years. Although files did not routinely contain assessments of family situations, we were able to obtain meaningful information for about a third of our subjects. In 70% of these cases marital discord, alcohol abuse, or violence was clearly documented. It is likely that omission of information for many inmates indicates a lack of problems, but at the least we have clear indication of early family problems in 25% of all cases.

There are other indications that subjects' criminality is at least partly attributable to their family histories. The median number of children in the family was 3.4, a bit high but not remarkable in itself. However, almost 30% of subjects had siblings who had been sentenced to a prison term; when we correct for those who were only-born children, the value becomes 32%. Of course, this may reflect either hereditary or environmental influences, or both, but it does indicate that criminal behaviors are related to family affiliation.

Personal History

Thus, within the context of our study, class differences seem to have relatively limited use in explaining criminal offenses later in life. The evidence here is rather indirect, but it is only a first examination of the role of background factors in the determination of criminal acts. Later, we will present other analyses that will strengthen our conclusion.

At the same time, we do not wish to argue that early experience is not important, for our data show some substantial effects of family history. We would expect that one's early experience is a major element in determining how one will react to events later in life. However, we would argue that abstractions such as social class have little direct effect on such learning, and that they will have little influence on later behavior in most cases. Of course, in environments where such factors are more strongly represented in individual experience, e.g., where there is stronger class consciousness and identification, the picture may be different.

If there is evidence of problems within our subjects' families, when we look at their own achievements and personal histories the problems are even more evident. Data in these areas are summarized in Table 3.4. For example, the average level of education achieved was 9.5 years of school, very close to previous estimates for the federal inmate population. However, the range was from grade 1 to university level, and 16% had completed no more than grade 8. Less than 20% had completed high school, and 45% had not completed grade 10, a level commonly used to assess competency for many sorts of employment. We also asked the age of leaving school, since inmates can raise their educational level in prison, and the data from

TABLE 3.4. Personal history measures of subjects (self-reports except where noted).

Variable	
Education and training	
Mean age left parents' home	17.3
Mean school grades completed	9.5
Job training (%)	
Professional or managerial	3.8
Skilled trade or equivalent	14.3
Semi-skilled trade or equivalent	50.4
Unskilled or none	31.6
Previous adjustment (%)	
Treated for psychological problems	1ö.8
Suicidal behavior	
Seriously considered suicide	29.3
Attempted suicide	12.8
Mention of alcohol problem in file	73.3
Relationships with women (%)	
Ever married	50.4
Never had relationship	9.0
Criminal history (from official files)	
Mean age at first offense on record	21.2
Percent 18 or under at first offense	54.7
Mean age at first prison term (excludes those with no previous imprisonment)	19.2
Mean total number of convictions	12.6
Percent total convictions	
1–3	20.5
4–9	23.6
10 or more	55.9

this measure strengthen the earlier impression: 10% had left school by the age of 14, and 30% left by the age of 16, percentages that are far higher than those for Ontario generally.

Lack of education was also reflected in job training and employment history. Only 18% had training for skilled, supervisory, executive, or professional occupations, and at the time they were arrested, only 14% worked at jobs in those categories. The largest single group, comprising 34%, had been unemployed, and half of those had never worked at a single job for as long as a year.

Thus, although social and economic indices showed only small differences from the general population for the aggregate of offenders we dealt with, personal histories were often characterized by major problems. As can be seen in Table 3.4, many had evidence of serious adjustment difficulties excluding criminal activities, e.g., alcoholism, suicide attempts, or serious emotional problems. As well, their development of long-term heterosexual relationships was often deficient.

With their levels of education and training, one would expect that many offenders would have had difficulties in establishing and maintaining stable places in society. However, we should not imply that their educational background was the cause of their criminal offenses. Rather, it appears that problems developed quite early in the lives of many subjects, as evidenced by the early onset of criminal careers and early difficulties in school. In these cases, delinquent behavior would have likely led to the deficiencies in education and training which we saw.

If we saw little evidence for the effect of original socioeconomic status on the development of criminal behavior, we can also say that most of our subjects showed positions in society that were socially and economically disadvantaged. However, much of this seems of their own doing. Many of them had achieved a substantial fall in social stratum from that of their origins, with job training and unemployment histories far worse than those of their fathers.

As we will see in the next chapter, there is much additional information to show the tenuous and unstable positions of many subjects within the social structure. If this is not predictable from socioeconomic factors, and offenders do sometimes drift downwards through social strata, we are led to ask how they manage to fall into this predicament. The answer which we will propose is that they are unable to cope adequately with life's ordinary challenges, and that they combine this with individual lifestyles that potentiate the likelihood of criminal behavior. The following chapters provide some details of both the argument and the evidence for it.

4
Lifestyle and Behavior on the Outside

In the first interview we spent much time gathering information about our subjects' behavior while they were living outside of prison. We had included a variety of questions about their activities, use of time, and relationships with other people, in an attempt to construct a picture of their lives and lifestyles.

These data for life on the outside cannot be considered as definitive, because they were gathered retrospectively. The reliability of recall is somewhat imperfect at best, with a good deal of distortion of memories over time. Since subjects had been arrested a median of about 5 months before the interview, there were likely some inaccuracies in what they remembered when we questioned them. In addition, some had spent relatively little time on the outside, at least in the period before their current term. Although our questions were intended to survey the 6 months prior to being arrested on the current charge, a few had not spent that long a period free since their release from a previous prison term, and in one or two cases we had to use periods as short as one month.

Time and Planning

Despite these problems, some interesting consistencies and regularities appeared in the results. Many subjects showed patterns of behavior that may be characteristic of a criminal lifestyle, but which are somewhat at variance with common perceptions about offender behavior.

One set of questions asked subjects to tell how much time they had spent in a variety of different types of activities, from sleep to socializing. We had tried to make the categories fairly exhaustive, so that we could account for most of the time in subjects' lives on the outside.

The average times spent on various activities are reported for each category in Table 4.1. The total time accounted for is about 25 hours daily, a difficult schedule even for those living fast-paced lives. The excess arises mostly because a given activity was sometimes counted in two categories.

TABLE 4.1. Summary of average time usage on the outside previous to current term of imprisonment.

Category	Mean daily hours
Sleep	7.0
Work, education or training	4.1
Socializing	4.3
Passive activity (TV, radio, recorded music)	3.8
Family activities and duties	3.3
Participatory activity (sports, hobbies)	1.1
Other	1.3
Total	24.9

For example, subjects often reported that they listened to music while they socialized, and this time might be counted twice. Given that we asked for time in each category independently of the others and without regard to the total, the total is gratifyingly close to 24 hours.

Therefore, we believe that these figures reflect reasonably accurately what our average subject did with his time. Regardless of the absolute accuracy of the numbers, the amounts of time in each category relative to the others are quite interesting. We can see that the greatest amount of waking time was spent socializing with friends. In contrast, somewhat less time was spent with families or in domestic tasks. A considerable amount of time was also spent in idle passive-spectator activities, almost as much as in working. Given the generally slow pace of activities, it is a bit surprising that the amount of time sleeping was at the low end of the average range; some 40% reported sleeping habitually at times during the day, so evidently our subjects did many of their reported activities at night.

The amount of time spent in all sorts of social activities is in contrast to the average amount of time spent working. As mentioned in chapter 3, just over one-third were unemployed, about four times the national unemployment rate at the time.

If we exclude the unemployed group, an average of just over 40 hours weekly was spent working. Thus, the low figure for daily work activity (averaged over 7 days) is the result of averaging the one-third of unemployed subjects into the totals. However, the high rate of socializing cannot be explained as the way the unemployed subjects found to fill their idle time, for even those who were employed reported much of their time spent in socializing. Employed subjects spent an average of 22% of their time in socializing, as compared to 25% for the unemployed, a difference that does not approach statistical reliability.

The impression of the pattern of subjects' lives that we get from time measures is reinforced by other sources of information, some of which are summarized in Table 4.2. In generating numbers and tables, we have imposed some order on subjects' time schedules. In their own thinking,

TABLE 4.2. Measures of planning and time use on the outside (self-reports).

Time framing	Percent
Living day-by-day (vs planning time)	82.9
Frequency of thoughts of future	
All of the time	10.0
Most of the time	23.1
Sometimes	28.5
Rarely	24.6
Never	13.8
Frequency of thoughts of present situation	
All of the time	22.1
Most of the time	21.4
Sometimes	24.4
Rarely	22.9
Never	9.2
Frequency of thoughts of the past	
All of the time	6.1
Most of the time	17.4
Sometimes	28.0
Rarely	35.6
Never	12.9

schedules or timetables did not have any relevance when they were living on the outside. Whether subjects were employed or not, for most of them there was little planning or anticipation of time, but rather a mode of living restricted to the present moment. Eighty-three percent said that they lived day by day and did not plan their time. We also had subjects rate the frequency with which they had thoughts of past, present, and future on a 5-point scale where 1 represented "all the time" and 5 was "never." The mean values were 2.8 for the present, 3.1 for the future, and 3.3 for the past. Many seemed to have been living in a perpetual present: the future would take care of itself and the past was stale news to be forgotten.

Did I plan my life or live day by day? Look, I always had something to do, and things happened all right without me worrying about them in advance. I mean, sometimes you could worry about something and it wouldn't even happen, so why worry about the future.

The past? The past is dead man, I never thought about it. Oh, once in a while I'd think about something good that happened to me before, like when my girlfriend and I were still together, but mostly I didn't care about it.

The distribution of time shown earlier in Table 4.1 fits well with this impression from the measures in Table 4.2 of how subjects organized—or did not organize—their time. The data generally suggest an average pattern that was somewhat loose and unstructured. Most subjects described passing their time rather than using it, in the company of others doing similar things.

Most of the time I would just find some of my buddies and we would maybe go to somebody's place and listen to some music or something. Sometimes I would bring a 26er (bottle of liquor) or maybe we would go to the hotel (tavern) for a while. I didn't drink much, just a few beers, but there wasn't much else happpening.

Sometimes I would go work on the car, I liked to keep it looking nice. In the evenings I would go to my old lady's house and we would do something. In the summer I liked to go fishing almost every day.

The picture of aimlessness is reinforced by other information gathered in the interview, most of which is summarized in Table 4.3. Most subjects had a network of friends with whom they spent their time. When we asked how many friends they had, the mean number reported was 5.0. Although most were not married, as will be discussed below, only 15% reported living alone, and even some of those were living in settings such as halfway houses. A small minority lived on their own, but most were anything but loners.

At the same time, living arrangements were frequently very imperma-nent, and many subjects moved around regularly. For example, 29% had been at their current addresses on the outside for no more than 6 months, and a total of 47% had been there no longer than a year. Some of this is attributable to a pattern of recidivism in which terms in prison are punctu-ated by occasional vacations to the outside world, but there were many who had been on the outside for several years but had never really estab-lished a fixed long-term residence.

Socialization

It is important to note that while subjects spent a great deal of their time in casual socializing, the relationships did not seem to be very close. Some subjects told us that they had felt that there was no one in whom they could confide when they had a problem, even though they spent most of their time with "friends." Relationships seemed to be generally fluid, with alliances often shifting within the context of a larger group.

In other ways, it seemed that subjects' emotional involvements often did not extend beyond the moment. If friends had a falling out one day, the next day the events would be forgotten. Once an event had occurred, it was no longer worth worrying about. Only acts that involved the world outside of the local social group, such as betrayal to the police, were not forgiven.

The tenuous quality of relationships can also be seen in looking at in-volvement with families. When asked to specify the individuals in their family, only 33% mentioned adult nuclear families, e.g., wives and chil-dren. But this does not imply any greater attachment to their families of origin, for the mean age at which they had left the home in which they were

TABLE 4.3. Measures of subjects' lifestyle and emotional states on the outside (self-reports except where noted).

Variable	Percent	Mean
Heterosexual relationships		
Currently married (legal or common law)	34.6	
Current relationship but unmarried	25.6	
Never had relationship lasting 6 months	15.0	
Socialization		
Number of friends		5.0
Proportion of friends in criminal activities		34.2
Proportion of acquaintances in criminal activities		49.8
Employment		
Working at time of offense	66.2	
At current job 6 months or less (excludes unemployed)	44.1	
Longest time job held ever (months)		38.4
Longest job ever no more than 6 months	41.4	
Means of support for unemployed		
Unemployment insurance and other gov't program	31.8	
Friends or family	15.9	
Criminal activities	40.9	
Living arrangements		
With family of origin	26.3	
With own nuclear family	49.6	
In nonfamily group arrangements	9.0	
Alone	9.8	
Mean time in current living arrangement (months)		75.6
Less than 6 months in current arrangement	28.8	
Emotions and life satisfaction		
Frequency of (weekly)		
Depression		2.6
Anger		2.6
Anxiety		3.4
Guilt		2.0
Never depressed	31.8	
Never angry	31.6	
Never anxious	29.3	
Never feeling guilt	50.4	
Satisfied with life on the outside	47.0	
Tried to make changes to improve life	48.2	
Had sleeping problems	23.5	

brought up was just over 17. Moreover, 52% claimed to have fathered children, but only 20% actually lived with their own children.

Similarly, a large proportion of our subjects showed some difficulties in forming and maintaining intimate personal relationships with women. Only about one-third said that they were married (either legally or common-law) at the time they were charged, and it was clear that many of these relationships were rather casual alliances.

When I got out from my last bit I ran into Linda. She had been living with a friend of mine who got sent to Millhaven, and then I moved in with her. So she said that we were married, and that was okay with me, and I really felt like a father to her children.

In addition to the men who said they were married, a further 26% reported a "relationship" with a woman, but 40% reported no current relationship at all. Of the entire sample, 15% had never had a relationship with a woman which lasted 6 months. We did check whether this might be owing to homosexual preferences, but only 3 subjects declared themselves as homosexual, even after being asked. Most of the rest cited unfavorable circumstances or lack of opportunities, but the most likely explanation was probably elsewhere. In the next chapter we will see that subjects' relationships with women were often rife with disagreements, quarrels, and even physical fights. From their descriptions of how they coped with the ordinary stresses of a relationship, we judged that many subjects lacked either the social skills to establish a relationship or the ability to sustain one on any reasonable reciprocal basis.

In summary, we can say that our typical subject lived an unstructured and unplanned life, with much dependence on a network of fluid and generally superficial relationships. There was evidence of instability in almost all aspects of their lives. For example, even if we exclude the unemployed, we find that almost half of the men had held their current job for no more than 6 months. If they changed jobs frequently, they also changed residences, activities, and even personal relationships.

At the same time, they were also stuck in the pattern of their changes, and there was little evidence of any interest in achieving a different lifestyle. As we will see later, subjects had a variety of problems in living outside, much as we all do, so they did not see the conditions they experienced as ideal. Still, about half said at the interview that they had been satisfied with their lives; of the others, very few had made any real efforts to change things. Even daydreams were not all that common, and 45% reported daydreaming rarely or never.

The retrospective reports we have on emotional states also indicate that most subjects had not been particularly unhappy with their lives. The mean reported frequencies of both anger and depression were 2.6 episodes weekly, with anxiety rates higher at 3.4 episodes weekly. While these values indicate that the average subject was far from placid, they also show no great amount of disturbance for most. Emotional responses may have been dulled by a high rate of drug and alcohol use, as we will see later, but the data seem to confirm that subjects had mostly reached some stability in their maintenance of a fluid and unstable lifestyle. Thus, the average pattern was one of casual, unplanned days, with greater dependence on friends than family or work, little focus, and no goals.

Criminal Activities

As one might expect, the loose lifestyle of the average subject was a likely facilitator for criminal activity. Interestingly, it appears that most of the criminal activities engaged in by our subjects were characterized by the same casualness as the rest of their lives. In their descriptions of their offenses we saw very little evidence of systematic planning or execution.

Criminal activities also took little time during the week, even for those subjects who considered themselves career thieves or burglars. We had included criminal activity in the "other" category of our time survey, but most of the things reported in this category were noncriminal in nature. When we specifically asked about illegal acts, many subjects readily admitted to a history of persistent offenses but said that little time was involved. Instead, most of their crimes seemed to be chosen and executed with the same casualness as their other activities. The myth of the master criminal matching wits with the police is as far from the truth as the paranoid visions of network television.

Well, I was sitting in the tavern with a friend, and then a guy he knew came over and started talking with us, and he said that he was going to pull a score on this warehouse, it couldn't miss. But I didn't like him too much so I said no, I mean he looked like a real goof to me. So anyway, he and Ronnie went to try it the next day, but they saw some lights on and they got scared away. The next day, Ronnie came and asked me again, and I had had a few beers so I said okay, what the hell. When we got there I didn't want to go in, so I told them I was going to stay outside. But then I heard a big noise and a lot of shouting so I ran in.

Certainly, the heavy emphasis on social contacts provided links to the criminal subculture. Half of the sample had close friends who were engaged in criminal activities (of course, often in the company of the subject). However, many offenses were committed with casual acquaintances rather than friends, much as most of us separate our friends from the people with whom we deal at work. Among the wider circle of acquaintances, the mean estimate was that 50% were involved in criminal behavior; only 22% of subjects said that none of their acquaintances were criminals.

While this shows a wide involvement in criminal activities, it also raises an interesting question. The typical lifestyle described here was generated from the aggregate of all subjects: it appears to fit a majority, and it also has considerable similarity with previous descriptions of criminal subcultures (e.g., Glaser, 1964; Irwin, 1970). However, a significant minority led lives that seemed much more stable and focused. For example, 31% of the sample had lived in the same residence for at least 5 years, 30% had maintained a continuing relationship with a woman for the same length of time, and, of course, 28% had never been convicted of any previous offenses that caused them to be sentenced to a prison term. Other measures show a similar number of exceptions to the generalized picture we draw here.

If this is so, then we are led to ask whether there is any relationship between the pattern of behavior described here and the occurrence of criminal offenses. In one aspect, this question cannot be answered from our data, for it asks to what extent individuals who show the pattern of behavior we have described are likely to commit crimes in the future. Since our data were retrospective, and since all subjects had already been convicted of a recent crime, this predictive relationship cannot be assessed.

However, it is possible to consider whether the various behaviors we have described are related to previous criminal records. As a measure of criminal history, we chose the total amount of time served in prison before the current term; we looked at the variety of measures we have discussed above to see if any were significantly related to previous imprisonment. Many were.

For example, there was good evidence that subjects who had not been previously imprisoned led more stable and settled lives. They had lived longer at their current addresses: 77 % had been there for at least 2 years, as opposed to only 20% of subjects who had been in prison for 24 months or more, a statistically significant difference ($\chi^2 = 27.8$, df = 4, $p < .001$). Similarly, 51% were currently married, in contrast to only 21% of subjects with 24 months or more of previous imprisonment ($\chi^2 = 9.2$, df = 2, $p < .01$). In addition, 16% of the no-prison group were unemployed, as compared to 40% for other subjects ($\chi^2 = 7.2$, df = 2, $p < .05$). Given this last result, it is not surprising that they also spent less time in social activities ($\chi^2 = 15.8$, df = 6, $p < .05$).

Some of these differences might be expected simply because individuals with long histories of imprisonment had probably not had the opportunity to establish long-term relationships, given the frequency with which their lives on the outside were interrupted by stretches of time in prison. Still, one cannot account for all of the differences in this way. Subjects without prior imprisonment were much more likely to have planned their time than the others ($\chi^2 = 9.1$, df = 2, $p < .02$). They had also achieved a higher level of education ($\chi^2 = 12.3$, df = 4, $p < .05$) even though they did not leave school any earlier. Even though they were more likely to have been working, they were less likely to say that they had problems in getting along with co-workers, ($\chi^2 = 11.5$, df = 4, $p < .01$). In short, they seemed generally better adjusted as well as more stable, and many of the differences do not seem to have much to do with the presence or absence of a history of previous imprisonment.

Thus, much of the pattern we see for our subjects' lives on the outside is associated with having been previously in prison. Many of the behaviors discussed here were not unique to this study, but we are able to see a more or less coherent picture of a lifestyle that seems to be characteristic of habitual offenders.

Where does this picture fit in the process of criminal offenses? We see two alternative lines of argument. The first is that certain lifestyles facilitate the occurrence of criminal acts. If a person leads the life we have described, his frequent socialization will likely bring him into contact with criminals, and his aimlessness may predispose him to accompany them in their activities. Of course, these factors alone are relatively weak determinants, and their effects must be considered in conjunction with other things, such as the coping problems discussed in the next chapter. However, when criminal activities do occur, then some time in prison may be the result, but on his release our man would likely return to his former life, with the same lifestyle, starting the cycle over again.

On the other hand, what we observe might be an effect of imprisonment. As we shall see, life in prison imposes a particular order on behavior. Some reasonable adaptations to the rules and regulations of prison life would be expected. We shall describe the sort of behaviors adopted by most prisoners in later chapters, but we may anticipate by saying that they are in many ways similar to the pattern we have described here. From this, it would be argued that prisoners adopt particular behaviors that are adaptive in prison, and that they maintain the same ways of reacting and behaving when they are released to the outside world. Thus, what we see here may be an indirect result of criminal behavior rather than a cause.

It is interesting to try to untangle the threads of inference from these two explanations, and the issues will arise repeatedly in the rest of this book. However, we should mention that reality is probably not so simple as we have made it appear here, for it may be the case that both sorts of processes play some role in the maintenance of criminal behavior. For example, evidence to be presented later is consistent with the claims that prisons strengthen or consolidate inappropriate ways of coping that are acquired on the outside, or that they stop the development of more effective behaviors that normally occurs on the outside.

While we can see the issues and arguments with the material in this chapter, it will be easier to understand and evaluate the various models of behavior after we have looked at the problems that offenders see in living outside of prison, and the ways they handle those problems. We do this in the next chapter.

5
Problems and Coping on the Outside

The Problems of Subjects

If we want to know how people deal with stressful situations, we must first identify those situations. Thus, as described earlier, we had included in our interview an extensive set of questions aimed at identifying the set of problems that each individual experienced in his life outside of prison. We ended up with up to 5 types of problems for each subject, described in his own words and ranked by him according to the perceived order of importance. The procedures we used were designed to ensure that each problem was really seen by the subject as having been significant.

We found that our offenders were able to specify their problems without much difficulty. By the time we had gone through the set of possible problem areas used as memory retrieval aids, there was usually a good deal of information. Only 2 of the 133 subjects claimed that they had had no significant problems on the outside. At the other end, only about one-sixth of the total specified 6 or more, indicating that our choice of 5 as a cutoff was fortuitous. The average number of problems included on the final lists was 3.8.

Interestingly, the great majority of listed problems were chronic rather than episodic. This may have occurred because it is easier to recall situations that persist over time, as opposed to single events, but it was probably also owing to the way we asked about situations. This may allow some interesting comparisons with other studies of coping that have concentrated on episodic events (e.g., Kanner, Coyne, Schaefer, and Lazarus, 1981).

After studying subjects' lists of problems we compiled a set of frequently mentioned problem categories, and then counted the number of subjects who listed a problem within each category. Since subjects had described problems in their own words, we had to judge whether a given item fit a category; in doing this, we chose to be conservative and did not count any case where there was a reasonable doubt about the fit. In a few cases, a subject had specified two closely related problems that fell within the same cate-

TABLE 5.1. Common problem categories on the outside previous to current term of imprisonment.

Category	Frequency of mention	Percent of subjects
1. Fights or arguments with wife or girlfriend	78	59
2. Money or financial difficulties	65	49
3. Conflicts with friends	52	39
4. Dissatisfaction with current lifestyle	45	34
5. Police or parole inquiries or restrictions	32	24
6. Loneliness or depression	30	23
7. Problems at work	27	20
8. Drug or alcohol use	18	14
9. Unemployment or unsuitable employment	16	12
10. Lack of future direction or goals	11	8

gory, e.g., conflicts with two separate co-workers; in these cases we counted the problem category only once.

The results showed that there was clearly some commonality across subjects in the problems they experienced. A listing of the 10 most commonly specified problems is shown in Table 5.1, with frequencies for each. A total of 74% of all the problems listed were included within the 10 categories shown, with 54% in the top 5 categories.

As can be seen, conflicts with heterosexual partners were the most frequent sort of problem, listed by a clear majority of subjects. About half mentioned some sort of financial difficulties. Frequencies for other problems ranged downward from these.

Interestingly, two of the top three categories are concerned with social relationships. In contrast, goal-related concerns were much less frequent. For example, items that fit the category of "lack of future direction or goals" were included by only 8%, and concerns with unemployment or underemployment were listed by only 12%. The latter figure is only a fraction of those who were actually unemployed, a finding that might be seen as inconsistent.

However, our problem-listing procedure was intended to measure what subjects perceived as significant problems in their lives, rather than our own assessment of their situations. If only one in three of the unemployed evaluated lack of work as a significant difficulty in their lives, then we see again subjects' relative lack of concern for anything beyond the immediate moment, especially when unemployment is contrasted with the importance for subjects of problems in social interactions. Thus, the data on problem frequency are nicely complementary to the conclusions in the preceding chapter.

Apart from these considerations, the assortment of problems that were related by each subject contained few items that were either surprising or unusual. Although we do not have comparable data for other populations, the most frequently cited categories seem common and ordinary. They are the sort of problems in living that we might expect to encounter in clinical practice, or, in less severe forms, to find in our own lives. Only one category on the list (number 5) is specific to people with criminal lifestyles or histories. Outside of prison, offenders must deal with the same sorts of problems as everyone else.

We also considered whether we could differentiate among subjects according to their problems. We looked first at the relationships between the number of problems on an individual's list and such variables as prior imprisonment, and the length of the current term. We could see no differences that even approached statistical reliability. Next, we looked to see if the inclusion of any particular problem was related to other variables. Here, we found only a few significant relationships: subjects with no prior prison experience were less likely to report a problem with co-workers, and they also listed problems with goals or the direction of their lives more frequently. However, these seem to be minor and isolated differences.

Although the problems a person perceives in his life may reflect his own individual concerns, they are also largely determined by external circumstances. We conclude that in general there is little that is unique or even special in the problems experienced by offenders while they live on the outside.

First Impressions of Coping

This study was conceived primarily as an analysis of how people respond to potentially stressful situations. From our theoretical perspective, we expected that most people would have more difficulty in dealing with unusual or especially hard conditions. However, for difficulties to arise it is not necessary for environmental conditions to be either out of the ordinary or unusually severe. What seems to differentiate maladaptive behavior from successful coping is primarily the way in which people respond to the problems they encounter, rather than the details of the problems. Poor coping ability can ensure that even simple everyday situations will become major sources of misery.

Therefore, it is not surprising that the problems that convicted offenders saw on the outside were generally mundane, and the similarity of immates' problems to the common lot only emphasizes the importance of looking at how they responded to life's circumstances. In this and the following sections, we will consider the information we received from our subjects on how they coped with life on the outside.

In chapter 2, we described in some detail the methods used in the interview to obtain information about coping behavior. The procedure required us to choose up to three problems from each subject's list for the coping analysis. For each of the problem situations chosen, we asked an extended series of questions in order to gather as much detail as possible about how the subject responded to his unique set of challenges.

Overall, subjects' reports gave us a strong impression that most of them had substantial deficiencies in the way they coped with problem situations. When faced with a problem, they usually attempted to deal with it directly and immediately, but their attempts were mostly unplanned, scattered, and impulsive, even though the problems were generally long-term and complex and needed some forethought, planning, and persistence.

When the initial attempts to solve a problem did not prove successful, the sequelae were not any better. The failure of a response to bring about some immediate improvement in the problem situation did not mean that it would be dropped, for repetition seemed to be more a matter of habit than the result of strategy. Some responses were used repeatedly, even though they were totally ineffective in remediating the problem, or were even harmful. Conversely, some behaviors that might have helped in the long run were dropped after a single half-hearted attempt to use them.

In short, we had the impression that coping was a disaster area for most subjects, and that only a few were really able to deal with life's problems with any degree of competence. We can best convey this by giving some typical examples of responses to the most common problems. Let us first consider one subject's set of responses to the most frequent class of problem described above, difficulties in relationships with wives or women friends.

(N.B. In this and other quotes to be presented, we have taken some liberties with respondents' actual utterances. Thus, we have omitted passages without indicating elisions, and sometimes we have also linked sentences that were spoken in answer to different questions. Comments or questions from the interviewer are summarized in parentheses.)

My wife wouldn't get motivated, she didn't clean the house. We had problems like that, and we fought a lot when I did drugs. I spoke to her about it sometimes, and she told me to stop bugging her, so I tried not to think about it. (What happened?) Well, I still was angry at her all the time. Sometimes I would go out and leave the house for the night, and then she would be happy to see me back, but she didn't do anything different. (More?) A couple of times we discussed it and she said that she would go out to work and I could do the housework. But she didn't have a job.

This case is representative of many others, showing scattered actions that were ultimately entirely ineffective in changing the original problem. This subject was typical of most whom we saw in that he was really trying to deal with his problems. The men we interviewed may have lacked the skill, persistence, and perspective to cope really effectively, but they were struggling, and in the end their efforts probably did them some good. However, the benefits were limited.

I was tired of the lifestyle (that he was leading), sick and tired of it all. (What did you do?) Nothing. I thought a lot and talked to my partner Bill. We decided we'd settle down for a while, but we never did. A few times I tried to look for a job, but it never worked. Sometimes, I'd go find a new lady for a few days. A lot of times I'd sit with my dog and tell him my problems, that way I'd feel better than after 5 hours with my wife.

My wife was unhappy about the friends I was going around with. (What did you do?) I told her not to bother me. Sometimes she would listen, but then she would start again and I would be mad. Mostly I would go for a stroll or a ride, or go and get my buddies and ride around, and we might get high. But when I went home she was still there.

Finally, there were a surprising number of cases in which the subject's responses probably made the situation worse.

The problem was that I was always fighting with my wife. When it happened I would go ride my motorcycle. Then I would pick up some friends and maybe go to the hotel and drink or get stoned on grass. I would wake up with good intentions but usually I got stoned and forgot about it. Sometimes I would stay away from the hotel for a few days, but eventually my friends would take me back there.

I was really jealous about my wife. I never knew she was fooling around for sure, but I thought she might be and I was really jealous. Sometimes I would do nothing, just sit back and let it go. Most of the time when I thought about it I would get drunk and just forget it for a while. I partied with younger people a lot, especially girls. I slept with a couple of girls, to get even with her. Once I took a crowbar and smashed the car of the guy I suspected (of being her lover).

We should emphasize that these responses were not unusual, but rather they were typical. Of course, responses differed across problems, because to some extent the problem determines the pattern of reactions that will occur. Nevertheless, we found the same gamut of ineffective, inappropriate, or exacerbating responses in every sort of situation. Subjects told us how they had given large parties to improve their mood when they were depressed from lack of money. Others, faced with demands to work harder on the job, decided to start arriving late for work, or assaulted the foreman, or just quit. One subject was anxious about memory loss from drug use, and another was worried about the chance of being caught for drug dealing: both handled their problems by getting stoned at every opportunity. The litany of poor coping we heard was long and varied. Worst of all it was consistent, for there were few exceptions to the rule of poverty.

Categories of Coping Responses

Although it was clear that our subjects had inadequate coping resources, we wanted to describe the results in a more systematic fashion. Therefore, we decided to classify and to quantify the obtained responses in a number of ways. We shall discuss the classification scheme in this section, and quantification in the next.

It is commonly assumed that the type of response one makes to cope with a stressful situation is a major determinant of one's success in dealing with the problem. For example, it is usually argued that people should be taught to face problems directly, rather than avoiding them or just seeking some relief for emotional distress. To examine modes of dealing with stress, we needed a typology of coping responses to categorize subjects' behavior.

Our first attempts at classification of coping behavior were based on other analyses in the literature, e.g., that of Lazarus. However, we found that these largely classified coping behaviors according to their intended functions or the motives they were supposed to express. When we were confronted with actual sets of responses it was often very difficult to divine the motive for a given response, and we found that many times the same response could be interpreted in several ways.

For example, a number of our subjects reported having struck their wives to deal with a disagreement. While our first impulse was to consider this a form of direct action, subjects also reported some reduction in their levels of emotional arousal after the assaults, so this behavior might also be classified as palliative, thus fitting two of Lazarus's major categories. We found similar uncertainty for many of the coping descriptions we had recorded, and there were many differences when more than one of us classfied the same responses. We concluded that the problem was in using a typology based on judgments of the motive or purpose behind responses. We could not judge these motives, and subjects themselves were often unsure, even if we asked them directly.

Therefore, we devised our own set of categories which classified behaviors according to their function in the situation, regardless of intentions or motives. The final list of the 11 types of response we arrived at is presented in Table 5.2. In practice, it is possible that a given response could have two closely related functions. For example, if a person leaves the scene of an argument to go talk with a friend, he is both escaping from the original situation and also seeking social support. One can get drunk to escape from an unpleasant situation, or to remediate an unpleasant emotional state, or just as a way of being with friends to get social support. In such cases, one cannot easily decide which function is primary. Thus, we allowed that a given response or set of responses could be tallied in several of our categories.

We wanted to see what sorts of responses each subject commonly used, but also to find out which modes were within their repertoire. Therefore, in scoring responses we adopted the strategy of crediting the use of as many categories as possible. We inspected the set of all responses reported by a subject for all of the situations examined in the interview, and parsed the list of categories to see if there was evidence of any behaviors within each mode. Thus, for each subject we generated a set of up to 11 categories for which he had demonstrated a capability of use.

The percentage of subjects who were judged to have shown responses

TABLE 5.2. Coping modes used on the outside previous to current term of imprisonment.

Category	Percent using
None (subject did not cope at all with problem; usually says that nothing could be done or that he was unable to act)	2
Reactive Problem-Oriented (attempts to deal with problem situation, but lacking evidence of persistence, planning, organization, or anticipation of future results)	100
Avoidance (staying away from situation in which problem occurs, or avoidance of thoughts about it)	46
Escape (physical removal of self from problem situation, or termination of thoughts about it)	30
Palliative (responses to reduce emotional distress from problem, most commonly by providing some contrasting pleasant event other than drugs or social support)	52
Social Support (use of others for comfort or reassurance, or sharing problems by self-disclosure)	32
Anticipatory Problem-Oriented (explicit recognition of nature of problem situation; systematic, organized and persistent attempts to resolve situation; evidence of planning and anticipation of future results)	13
Reinterpretive Re-evaluation (changes in appraisal or perception of situation to reduce perceived threat)	7
Reinterpretive Self-control (use of self-control techniques to reduce, redirect, or otherwise alter emotional response to situation, thus reducing threat)	10
Anticipatory Substitution (deliberate choice of behaviors incompatible with occurrence of problem situation, generally using strategy of filling time)	12
Alcohol or Drug Use (ingestion of substances for purpose of relieving emotional distress or to dull awareness of problem)	64

within each category is shown in Table 5.2. As can be seen, there were large variations across modalities in the frequency of use. Therefore, we shall discuss the categories each in turn in the following sections.

REACTIVE PROBLEM SOLVING

Certainly the most common sort of response we found was the one we have categorized as reactive problem solving. On the basis of previous analyses that differentiated direct attempts at problem solving from other modes such as avoidance or palliation, we had expected that inmates might often fail to attempt to deal with their problems at all, but this was not the case. Every subject reported some sort of attempts to deal directly with at least some of his problems, and in general it appeared that offenders almost always attempted to solve their problems at some time.

Responses in this category took many forms, some of which can be seen in the examples presented earlier. For example, interpersonal problems were met most commonly by some attempts to talk things out. Worries about personal limitations, e.g., drinking problems or an uncertain future, usually led to a resolve to reform and do better.

These behaviors are certainly in the right direction, but from asking subjects about the consequences of their actions we know that such responses were rarely of much use in resolving problems. This is not surprising, for each when subjects knew what sort of actions were required they lacked the skill to execute them successfully. When they tried to discuss interpersonal problems, they usually confronted rather than negotiated; when they resolved to change, they neglected the means of doing so. Without the means, even the best resolve is of little benefit, as most of us know from our attempts to reform our offenses against ourselves, e.g., habitual dieting or smoking recidivism. Still, if these offenders were not skilled in solving their problems, at least they were actively struggling with them.

As we have already pointed out, these attempts to deal with problems were almost always lacking in planning, organization, or persistence. They are best described as reactive because they occurred in reaction to each occasion on which a problem was evident, without any anticipation of the next occurrence.

OTHER LOW-LEVEL COPING MODES

When they were not attempting to deal with problems directly, subjects often employed a number of other ways of mitigating the stress induced. These include categories we called avoidance, escape, palliation, and social support. While we would consider them to be basically low-level coping strategies, they can be effective in dealing with problems, but remediation is only temporary because these strategies leave the basic situation unchanged.

Avoidance and escape are very similar, both resulting in a separation between the problem and the individual. We had allowed for avoidance and escape either from the actual situation (physically leave the field) or from thoughts ("put it out of my mind"). However, outside of prison we found that the separation was almost always physical, as, for example, in subjects' reports that they had walked out on arguments (escape) and then stayed away from the scene to forestall a renewal (avoidance).

Altogether, the majority of subjects showed use of either escape or avoidance. Sometimes their actions showed some planning, for example when a subject left the city to get away from his problems or went camping to "do something totally different." Usually they involved at least a little forethought, as when a subject stayed in his room to avoid confrontations with another family member, or skipped work to avoid a troublesome coworker. However, use of escape or avoidance did not seem to be the result of reflecting on how best to deal with a problem.

Seeking social support was another kind of coping response, used by about one-third of the sample. Given the high rate of socialization seen on the outside, one might have expected more. However, it appears that subjects socialized for the rewards it provided in itself and as a way of passing time. The macho image they often felt compelled to adopt in public made it difficult for them to discuss their problem with associates, and they often explicitly mentioned that they did not feel able or willing to confide in the people with whom they spent the greatest part of their time. Consistent with this was the fact that when they did seek social support it was almost always from their wives or other family members. There were probably as many who sought comfort in their pets as who brought their personal problems to their "friends" for advice or succor.

The last of the low-level categories was that involving the use of palliative measures to improve emotional states. Over half of our sample specified particular things that they sometimes did to improve their mood when they had a problem. For any individual, there seemed to be a small number of favorite activities which were used as palliatives, but overall there were a great variety. Physical activities such as walking were commonly used: some walked in the city for stimulation, others walked in the country for the quiet, others just walked for the pleasant effects of muscular exertion. Interestingly, more strenuous exercise or sports were hardly mentioned at all; as we shall see, this is in contrast to what we find inside prison. Other commonly used palliatives included listening to music, riding around in cars or on motorcycles, or just relaxing in the sun. However, some subjects cited more unusual activities such as deliberately smashing things (usually someone else's) or spending money (even if they hadn't any to spend).

There is, of course, nothing wrong with the use of what we call low-level modes of coping. Almost all of us employ them from time to time, because they provide some effective relief from the pressure of daily problems, even if it is only short-term and temporary. Most of us need to concentrate our attention and efforts on one problem at a time, and this often means deferring thoughts of other problems: you can't worry about the bats you discover in the attic when you go up to fix the leaking roof, at least not until the roof is fixed or the rain stops. Likewise, we can often get some helpful advice, or at least sympathy, when we share our problems with others (indeed, one can teach people to "pass it on" as an effective therapeutic technique). And the use of good palliatives is an effective way of dealing with some of fortune's more outrageous slings and arrows; it has even been shown that palliation might be a prophylactic against depression (Rippere, 1979).

Rather, we see it as insufficient to use these short-term strategies excusively, without any efforts aimed at long-term or permanent remediation of chronically difficult situations. Sometimes this is unavoidable even in a normal environment, for some problems are insoluble. For example, grief after the loss of a loved one is inevitable, and it cannot be resolved but only palliated until the passage of time grows a layer of scar tissue over the wound. However, the majority of our everyday problems can be improved on a long-term basis or even removed entirely if we cope well enough. The person who does not work to resolve those problems that are amenable to change is likely to have things accumulate until they wear him down or break him. At that point, maladaptive behavior will likely result.

Thus, we consider that the coping modes we have already discussed are very useful, but that there will likely be problems when a person uses them exclusively. From the data we have, we calculated that at least 35% of our subjects fell into such a category, that is, they used only the categories considered above. Thus, we again have evidence of limitations in the coping abilities of many subjects.

HIGHER-LEVEL COPING MODES

We can see more of the same when we look at the remaining response categories. The next four modes of coping shown in Table 5.2 are what we consider to be higher-level strategies. They all involve some active thinking about one's situation, and generally require planning and analysis. Our categories include the sorts of techniques that are taught by contemporary cognitive therapists (e.g., Meichenbaum, 1977; Ellis and Grieger, 1977) to people who are having trouble dealing with the problems of everyday life. However, this does not mean that their use is restricted, for we would expect that they are the sort of things that the majority of people do without special training.

None of these coping modes were used by more than a small minority of the offenders we interviewed. Even when problems were solvable, subjects almost always restricted their efforts to the reactive behaviors discussed above. Very few of them ever made any systematic effort to analyze a problem, to consider alternatives, or to redefine or reevaluate their situations. Instead, they endured their difficulties, thus perpetuating them.

ALCOHOL AND DRUG ABUSE

In the process of classifying coping, we were presented with one final type of response which could not be ignored, namely the use of alcohol or other drugs. On the basis of the extant literature and from our previous experience, we had expected that substance use—and abuse—would be widespread among offenders. Therefore, we had included some questions about it in the interview, and a questionnaire was devised to get detailed quantitative information about usage.

We had also expected that instances of drug and alcohol use could be classified into one of the other 10 coping categories, as either ways of escaping or as palliatives. However, our findings made this difficult, for the occurrence of substance abuse was so common and so widespread as to overwhelm our expectations.

In some cases the data did show clear instances where alcohol or drug use was just a behavior used in coping, and could fit into one of the other categories:

What did I do when my wife left? I went out and started drinking, and I didn't stop until I couldn't remember what had happened. (Escape)

I didn't know where I was going or whether I could get out of the mess I was in. I sat around for a day just getting depressed, and then I said "This is stupid, if you can't change it, you can't change it." So I decided to make myself feel good. I went out and scored some reds and spent three days popping them. When they were gone I was really wasted, but I felt better. (Palliative)

However, in many other cases it appeared that drinking and use of other drugs were so endemic in subjects' lives that they could not easily be tied to specific problems, or to coping, or really to anything else. They were pervasive and omnipresent.

Did I drink to stop thinking about my problems? Hell, I drank in the morning, I drank at night. Sometimes I drank so much I couldn't remember drinking. Maybe drinking was my problem, I don't know. But I didn't drink to forget or to escape or to do anything, I just drank.

Because of this difficulty, we considered instances of alcohol or drug use as a final category of coping responses. This category differs from the others in that it was often not tied to specific problems, but nevertheless it may be seen as a response to an individual's life situation as a whole.

We can see from the responses to the coping questions that a substantial majority of subjects did use drugs in reaction to their problems, at least sometimes. Most often used was alcohol, but cannabis was also common and a wide variety of other drugs were mentioned.

For more information on drug use we can turn to the results from our questionnaire, as summarized in Table 5.3. Alcohol use was, of course, the greatest among all the drugs included, and virtually all subjects reported drinking alcoholic beverages at least occasionally. In good Canadian taste, beer was the most preferred drink, followed by spirits, with only a minority ever drinking wine.

What is impressive is the total amount of reported drinking. For the entire sample, the mean number of drinking days was 15.1 per month. We had set a month as equal to 4 weeks or 28 days to equate across time units, so this figure represents something over a majority of days. One-quarter of all subjects reported that they drink every day.

In order to measure the amount of alcohol consumed, we converted the reported amounts into standard units, where one unit equals one 12-ounce bottle of beer (it should be remembered that Canadian beer contains about

TABLE 5.3. Alcohol usage on the outside (from drug use questionnaire).

	Percent	Mean
Reported drinking alcohol	91.0	
Choice of beverages[a]		
Beer	74.4	
Liquor	61.7	
Wine	28.6	
Frequency of drinking (including nondrinkers)		
Mean frequency (per 28-day month)		15.1
Drink on majority of days	47.4	
Drink daily	24.8	
Drinks per drinking occasion		
Mean total		14.8
Over 6	71.4	
Over 12	42.8	
Daily amount of drinking (frequency x amount)		
Mean units all subjects (including nondrinkers)		8.0
Over 6 units daily	47.2	
Over 12 units daily	34.0	
Connection with principal offense		
Used alcohol on day of offense	57.9	
Considered selves "drunk" at offense	30.1	
Said alcohol contributed to offense	35.3	

[a]Total exceeds 100% because of use of multiple beverages.

5% alcohol) or a 1.5-ounce shot of spirits, or a 5-ounce glass of wine. As can be seen in Table 5.3, the mean amount consumed per drinking session was very high, enough to produce substantial intoxication even in the most experienced or habitual drinkers. Over 70% of drinkers averaged at least 6 units per session, a level commonly used as evidence of alcohol abuse.

When we combine the frequency of drinking with the amount per session to generate an overall estimate of alcohol usage, we arrive at a figure of 8.0 units consumed daily for all subjects. Although this figure is inflated because of the contribution of the heaviest drinkers, it shows the impressive size of the problem that the correctional system must deal with. We estimate that about half of the sample was in need of treatment for alcohol abuse: in addition to the overall average, 47% of subjects averaged more than 6 units daily, and 34% averaged at least 12 daily. At these levels of consumption, permanent damage and deterioration are almost inevitable after a year or two.

Not surprisingly, alcohol use was also associated with subjects' criminal offenses. A total of 58% reported drinking on the day of their most serious or index offense, and 30% described themselves as drunk at the time of the offense. These figures must be taken cautiously, since some inmates may have wished to diminish their responsibility by attributing their crimes to alcohol. At the same time, the results are quite consistent with all of the

TABLE 5.4. Frequency of drug use.

Drug	Percent			
	Used ever	Use daily	Use weekly[a]	Frequency of use (month)[b]
Alcohol	99	25	88	16.6
Cannabis	81	23	62	15.5
Speed, amphetamines	39	8	20	7.8
Opiates	20	6	11	10.7
Cocaine	32	2	12	3.5
Hallucinogens	35	2	13	3.7
PCP	21	2	4	1.4
Tranquilizers	35	10	21	10.9
Solvents	5	1	1	1.3
Others	3	—	1	1.0

[a]Four times monthly or greater.
[b]Frequencies for users only.

other evidence on alcohol use, and may even be an underestimate given that several subjects declined to discuss the circumstances of their offenses.

If our figures on alcohol use show a problem greater than previously documented for the Canadian system, they are in agreement with data from elsewhere (e.g., Myers, 1982, found levels for British offenders that were slightly higher than ours, but still fairly close when comparable groups are considered). However, previous surveys have looked at use of either alcohol or other drugs. Because we wanted to examine problems in adaptation as much as possible, we included both.

Although alcohol was certainly the greatest problem drug, there was also evidence of abuse of a great variety of other substances. Second to alcohol was cannabis, as would be expected from its frequency of use in the general population. Eighty-one percent of our sample reported having used cannabis at some time, with 34% using it on at least half of all days and 23% using it daily. These numbers are lower than those for alcohol use, but comparing amounts of consumption is impossible because we are not able to estimate intake of the active ingredients in cannabis from a survey. (However, there seems again to be an association with offenses, as 38% reported use of cannabis on the day of their principal offense, and 20% said that they were "high" at the time of the offense.)

In addition, substantial proportions of the inmate sample had used a variety of other drugs. Table 5.4 shows a summary of the data. Out of the 8 classes of drugs shown in the table, the mean number used was 2.7, with a range from 0 to all 8.

Thus, the amount of abuse of both alcohol and other drugs by the subjects in this study was quite considerable. As an overall measure of drug use, we calculated a drug frequency index, which was the sum of the monthly frequencies of use for each of the 10 drug categories, regardless of the amount on any occasion. Using a simplified 28-day month, the index thus had a possible range of from 0 to 280. The median value was 28.4, indicating that the majority of subjects used one substance or another at least daily. For some, the problem was much greater, with 26% having index values over 56 and up to 100, that is, using more than two drugs daily.

While some of the reports may have been exaggerated, there can be no question that drug use was at a high level in our sample. When we add this to the information about alcohol use, we can see that the total problem is almost catastrophic, and it is certainly larger than what can ever be treated with the programs and facilities currently available in the Canadian federal system. Alcoholism ought not to be considered separately from other drugs, for a great many offenders are polydrug abusers: several times we heard statements like, "I took anything I could get, whenever I could get it."

This leads us to believe that many offenders are generally maladaptive. We see problems in coping, alcoholism, and, of course, also in the occurrence of criminal behavior. The causal interrelations of all of these are very interesting, and we shall consider them later.

INSIGHT

We wanted to find out not only how subjects actually had coped with their problems but also how well they were capable of coping in favorable circumstances and how much insight they had about their difficulties in coping. Therefore, we had included in the interview questions asking for subjects' evaluations of their own coping and for their perceptions of any possible relationships between their behavior and subsequent difficulties.

The first type of question was included in the coping inquiry. After finding out what subjects had done to deal with a problem, we asked them to look back and tell us what would have been the optimal response in the situation. The results from this question were sparse. The majority of subjects simply said that the most appropriate things were exactly what they had done. When the answer differed from this, it usually varied only in the intensity or persistence of efforts to resolve the problem, without any details. For example, if a subject was discussing an unemployment problem he might say that the best thing would have been to "keep looking for work" until he found it, or if the problem was his relationship with his wife he would say that he "should have worked it out."

We had also included a series of questions asking about subjects' perceptions of the relationship between their problems and their criminal offenses. The results were not very helpful, and they added very little to our understanding of the processes involved in the occurrence of criminal offenses. Often we had to repeat the questions, as though they were unusually difficult or posed in a foreign language. Equally often, we ourselves found it difficult to interpret the answers.

Certainly there were indications that some of the responses to problems that we had heard, such as substance abuse, were associated with criminal offenses for many subjects. A total of 58% reported drinking on the day of their most serious offense, and 30% described themselves as drunk at the time of the offense. These figures may even be an underestimate, given that several subjects did not accept the official version of their offense and declined to discuss the circumstances. However, when we asked about possible relationships between alcohol and their offenses, they were mostly unclear as to the connection. A few said that the disinhibiting or dulling effects of alcohol had caused their offense, but almost as many said that the connection was that they needed money from crime to buy more alcohol. Others said that they were sure that alcohol was connected to their crimes, but that they could not tell us how. In the end, we decided that most of these admissions owed more to the wish to shift some of the blame to Demon Rum than to any insight about the determinants of behavior.

We might conclude that our questions in these areas were unclear or poorly phrased. However, on reviewing them ourselves they appear reasonably simple and straightforward, and we believe that the answers show rather the limitations of subjects' understanding of their own behavior. Not only had they dealt poorly with their problems, but they did not know better ways to respond. As they had lived without planning or direction, so had they created for themselves a major part of their difficulties without realization. In all, they demonstrated a notable lack of insight about the causes of their problems or the limitations of their ways of handling them.

The Quality of Coping

We have some (largely impressionistic) evidence that our subjects were unable to cope satisfactorily with common and ordinary situations. However, impressions can be mistaken. To be convincing, one needs to show a sizable portion of the original material on which the impression is based. We have given some examples here, but only enough to communicate some of the flavor of the responses, and the reader must take it on faith that the chosen examples are fairly typical. Therefore, we decided that it was essential for us to quantify what we observed. Quantification was also important because we wanted to relate coping ability to some other behaviors, and in particular, to see how it could be used to predict some criteria of adaptation.

One way of quantifying the data was to code responses into the categories which we have just described. This allowed a more precise and detailed description of the response process, and it is the principal approach to quantification taken by previous researchers in the area. As they have done, we assumed some hierarchy of good or effective coping across the various categories, roughly the order in which we discussed them (with the exception of drug-taking). Thus, we would say that someone who employs a strategy of anticipatory problem solving is coping better than another person who avoids facing the problem.

However, the classification technique has some limitations that make it unsatisfactory as a way of evaluating coping. In the first place, situations can constrain the range of available actions. For example, as we shall see later, many of the problems that men experience in prison are in principle insoluble: they can be coped with, but they cannot be resolved because they are inherent in the conditions of contemporary prisons. In such cases, a person who used modes of coping less powerful than that of systematic problem solving may be doing the best that is possible under the circumstances. If coping is being assessed, he ought to be judged in terms of what things are possible given the constraints of the situation. Previous work has been more concerned with absolute classification rather than relative evaluations of coping.

However, there is a more serious problem in attempting to use a category system as a measure of the quality of coping. One can use a type of response well or badly. If we are interested in measuring how well people cope, we can easily be misled by a category system, for the use of a given category is counted whatever the quality of the response within the category. For example, we found that some subjects went to ask help from family members, unburdening themselves of their problems and seeking advice; others just used their families as convenient places to express their anger or frustrations; still others sought the company and communicated very little. Yet, each of these were classified as cases of seeking social support.

If we consider that the purpose of coping behavior is to alleviate the distress from problems, then we ought to be evaluating responses in terms of their efficacy in reducing that distress, both present and future. Looking at it this way, we must consider not only what one does in a situation, but also how well one does it. Thus, we worked out scales and procedures for rating the efficacy of coping, independent of other categories.

We set up two rating scales. The first measured the positive effects (benefits) that the behavior in a situation would likely produce, both on the person's emotional state and on the problem itself. The second scale assessed possible or likely deleterious effects (risks or costs) of the same behavior. Since we wanted to measure the overall efficacy of a person's coping, ratings were made only for the entire set of responses reported by each individual for each problem. Considering how the possible responses in a situation are constrained by the circumstances, estimates of efficacy using the benefits scale were always made relative to the responses possible in that situation. After ratings were made for the responses to each prob-

TABLE 5.5. Coping benefits and costs rating scales.

Description	Score
1. Benefits	
An optimal response:	5
Long-term and general remediation of problem situation, and/or relief of emotional distress is likely.	
Generally effective:	4
May provide some long-term partial remediation or relief, or short-term general remediation or relief; however, could be improved.	
Some usefulness:	3
Short-term and partial remediation or relief is likely, but responses have substantial limitations.	
Ineffective action:	2
Some action is apparent, but very little remediation or relief is likely.	
None:	1
Either no action, or action is unrelated to problem and provides no likely remediation or relef.	
2. Risks or costs	
None	4
Minor risk or cost:	3
Short-term exacerbation.	
Major risk or cost:	2
Short-term major exacerbation or long-term minor exacerbation.	
Extreme risk or cost:	1
Long-term and major exacerbation; catastrophic outcome likely.	

Note. For these scales, the entire set of responses for each problem is given a single rating. Rating is in terms of the overall probable benefits (costs) of a response set toward the relief (exacerbation) of emotional distress consequent on a problem situation, and/or removal or remediation (worsening) of the problem situation itself.

lem, they were combined and averaged across problems for each subject, to yield overall scores for individuals.

Data from the coping benefits and risk scales were considered separately, but for most purposes a single efficacy score was generated by multiplying the values from the two scales for each subject. Descriptions of the rating scales are given in Table 5.5.

In practice, these scales were not difficult to use. For example, here is a set of responses that was considered optimal and was assigned a benefits score of 5:

Well, I got onto welfare and my mother gave me some money, but I didn't want to take it from her. So I got the newspaper and started looking for jobs. Then I made the rounds of the guys I knew and told them I was looking, maybe they could help. I must have filled out 30 applications, every place I could think of. (More?) I kept telling myself, "Things will get better, I can wait it out." Sometimes I didn't believe it and got really down, but the next day I was back at it. So finally I landed a job in (. . .) and it paid okay but after a week I realized that it was a dead end. (What did you do?) I decided that I couldn't do better without any training, so I started a course at the local college, I could do it at night while I kept my job.

In contrast, the following set of answers received a rating of 3:

When I got out I had a job lined up but I quit after a week because the boss was on my case a lot. Then I was on the pogey (unemployment insurance) for a while. I went to the unemployment office a couple of times but there wasn't much there. (More?) When I had money I'd go to the tavern and have a few beers. I didn't think about the problem that much, because there wasn't much I could do about it. (More?) Well, after a while I started little jobs to get some extra money. (What kind of jobs?) You know houses, break-ins.

While this answer shows some behaviors that might be helpful, they were not systematically or persistently practiced. It should be noted that they included some criminal activity as a way of getting money. We considered that this was at least somewhat effective, and rated criminal behaviors the same as any others. Thus, a bank robbery might receive a rating of 3 or 4, depending on the amount of money stolen. Of course, these behaviors also received nonzero values on the risk scale, which would drop the combined efficacy scores a great deal.

Reliabilities with these same rating scales for similar material had been calculated before (Porporino, 1983). For two raters, the reliabilities had varied from .77 to .97 for single problems, with a combined reliability of .95 for the average of 6 problems. In this study, the selection of problem situations was different, so we repeated the checks. The coping responses obtained for problems within prison at the first interview were rated by both authors. Reliabilities for the efficacy scores were .89, .86, and .86 for the first, second, and third problems listed, respectively. The mean efficacy scores across problems for the two raters correlated .85. This suggests that the efficacy of coping responses can be scored consistently by experienced independent raters.

The results from the rating scales confirm and extend the conclusions from the other ways of assessing coping. Again, one is struck by the overall poor level of coping in response to problems in outside life. On the benefits scale, the mean rating for all subjects was 2.36. Since the scale runs from 1 to 5, this indicates a level of effectiveness only just above "entirely ineffective" and somewhat below "of some limited use."

Comparable studies for the general population are not available, although a study by Haley (1983) found a mean value of 4.0 using the same scale to measure coping in a group of university students. In any case, the scores given here provide another demonstration of the deficiencies in coping among offenders.

The case is further strengthened when we consider the results of the risks scale. A score below 4 on this scale indicates that a subject responded in a way that might increase the deleterious effects of a problem, or exacerbate the problem itself. For example, attacking someone with whom one was having a disagreement would be considered a minor risk; attacking them with a weapon would present a major risk.

Seventy percent of subjects had a score indicating a significant risk for at least one of their problems. If we consider only the single problem considered most serious by the subject, 54% had risk scores assigned, that is, they responded to their most serious problem in ways that would ordinarily result in making it worse.

Some of these risk scores were assigned because of criminal behaviors that subjects had committed in attempts to deal with their problems, for example robberies or assaults. However, most of the responses that were judged as presenting nontrivial risks were not specifically criminal in nature. An appalling number of subjects reacted to common situations in counterproductive ways, e.g., reacting to perceived wrongs by deciding to "get even," or avoiding troubling thoughts by taking large amounts of drugs habitually. If anything, the assigned scores underestimate the extent of counterproductive coping responses, for there were many other similar behaviors that were not serious enough to cause the assignment of a risk score. For example, one inmate had a disagreement with his wife over whether or not to have children, and then refused to talk with her about anything.

Clearly, the men we interviewed had shown a lack of foresight in considering the likely consequences of their actions, and as a result they were often their own worst enemies. If their original problems were not necessarily of their own making, their responses to the original situations often played a large part in producing the extraordinary final circumstances in which they sometimes landed.

Thus, from all of the analyses we performed we are led to conclude that most subjects had a great deal of trouble coping with life outside of prison. They were poor at adopting responses that could ameliorate their problems, and they had an inadequate repertoire of effective coping responses, especially the higher-level strategies that might provide long-term or general improvement in their situations. Often they responded in habitual, inappropriate, or stereotyped ways, despite the nature of the problem.

With the data from the risks scale we see how they often increased their difficulties by the behaviors that they chose, and one could predict that they would enlarge their everyday problems into a quicksand of maladjustment. It is not surprising that many had shown evidence of maladjustment before, other than their troubles with the law, and many other measures show this. For example, 13% reported that they had made a serious attempt at suicide, and 28% had been in institutions other than prisons, mostly psychiatric treatment centers. From the evidence we have on their coping, we would have predicted that some sort of major maladaptive consequences were almost inevitable for many: if they had not committed criminal offenses and been imprisoned, some other calamitous events might have occurred.

On the other hand, some subjects managed to cope reasonably well. For example, efficacy ratings were fairly evenly distributed throughout their range, and we would estimate that over 10% of the sample showed superior coping ability. Therefore, it will be possible to consider what factors are associated with good and bad coping, even within the population of criminal offenders. Such analyses are presented later.

Relationships Between Measurement Types

The three sources of data we have considered above—lifestyle variables, qualitative categorization of coping, and quantitative evaluations of coping —all show convergence on a picture of inadequate ways of dealing with problems. The question was, are the data actually showing the same picture from different perspectives, or do they reveal different behaviors. This question led us to look at the relationships among the different measures. We calculated correlations between the overall coping efficacy measure and most of the other measures we have considered in this chapter.

The results can be seen in Table 5.6. A variety of variables in several categories are correlated with coping efficacy, although most of the correlations are fairly small. However, if we disregard the size of the relationships, we can see that the set of variables that correlate with coping ability includes many of the same measures that appeared to characterize the lifestyle of offenders on the outside.

For example, we can see that poor coping is associated with instability, as measured by such things as lack of relationships with women and mobility in residence. Poor coping is also associated with relatively high proportions of time in socializing and passive activities, and low proportions in work and directed activities. Similarly, there are correlations with variables measuring how people frame time: poor coping is associated with lack of planning and infrequent thoughts of the future.

The other class of variables prominently associated with coping is comprised of those measuring previous criminal histories and affiliation with a criminal subculture. Thus, men who might otherwise be defined as core offenders, with offenses at a young age and many previous offenses, have poor coping ability, at least as we have assessed it.

With the given pattern of correlations, there is one possible flaw in our method. We have observed that coping efficacy is correlated with both lifestyle and criminal history. If these are related to each other, then the observed correlations between coping and criminality may be only an indirect reflection of the relationship between lifestyle and criminality. Therefore, we recalculated the correlations between coping and criminality, using partial correlation techniques that control for the effects of the lifestyle variables. Although the resultant values are generally lower than those shown in Table 5.6, the differences are minimal and significance levels are unchanged. Thus, coping and lifestyle measures are each independently related to criminal history.

TABLE 5.6. Correlations with coping on the outside previous to the current prison term.

Variable	Correlation
Lifestyle	
Marital status	.18*
Time in current residence	.18*
Longest relationship with a woman	.17*
Plan or live day by day	.39***
Proportion of time:	
Working	.26**
Socializing	−.21*
Passive activity	−.18*
Participatory activity	.22**
Frequency of thoughts of the future	−.20*
Frequency of anger	−.15*
Frequency of guilt	−.18*
Criminality	
Age at first recorded adult offense	.34***
Number of convictions	−.39***
Total time of previous imprisonment	−.34***
Percent of acquaintances criminals	−.20*
Visible tattoos	−.32***
Current sentence length	.24**
Background	
Social class	.19*
Number of siblings	−.21**
Coping history	
Previous psychological problems	−.18*
Drug frequency index	−.29**
Alcohol abuse index (days 6+ units)	−.33***
Life Events Scale	−.15*
Total number of problems cited	.04

*$p<.05$
**$p<.01$
***$p<.001$

After the above two classes of variables, the other measures significantly correlated with coping efficacy are expectable. These include mostly specific indications of poor coping, such as high rates of drug and alcohol use. However, it is interesting to note some things that appear not to be related to assessed efficacy. Most prominently among them are measures of whether an individual used each of our respective coping categories, demonstrating that there is some disjunction between the type of response to a situation and the effectiveness of that response. That is, as we discussed before, what matters is not how one responds but rather how well. The only exceptions are more or less artifactual: drug use often lowered efficacy ratings because it was seen as a risk factor, and in assigning scores we had considered systematic problem-oriented responses to be better than other modes of responding.

Background factors were mostly unrelated to coping, although the relationships with social class and family size are interesting. Moreover, coping did not relate to any measures we had of subjects' current problems. The presence of any particular problem, or even the total number of problems, is not related to the ability to deal with problems. This reinforces our earlier conclusion that stressors in offenders' lives are not especially unusual and not strongly related to their offenses.

Some Hypotheses

We are struck by the convergence of the results from the different ways we have used to describe the behavior of our subjects on the outside. We find that there is a common lifestyle, and that it is associated with previous criminal careers. At the same time, both the criminality and the lifestyle are associated with poor coping ability. We can predict that the more a person has been in prison, the more like other ex-inmates will be his behavior on the outside, and the more problems he will have in living on the outside.

This raises the question of causality. Do prisons produce poor coping? We shall consider this question later when we have adduced some additional evidence, but before anything else we must admit that our data will not lead to any definitive answer. We saw subjects only after a long and tangled process, so that even if there had been any simple determinative link it would have been lost in a distant behavioral past. Even more, we would expect that any process operating here would be interactive, so a simple linkage at any time would be unlikely. Thus, the question may be unanswerable (unless one could actually carry out a longitudinal study in which every young man of a generation was followed for at least several years).

However, it is possible to delineate some alternatives that would fit the linkage we see between poor coping, lifestyles, and a history of offenses and imprisonment. The first explanation is that prisons change people so that they are less able to cope with a free environment. As we shall see, the special conditions of imprisonment facilitate some ways of coping and make others difficult. We could hypothesize that prisons teach people ways of acting which they retain after release, and that the behaviors learned in prison are maladaptive on the outside. Thus, the men who have spent the most time in prison would be the worst adapted on the outside.

While we cannot test this directly, it generates some testable predictions. If offenders cope poorly on the outside, it is because prisons have damaged them by training inappropriate responses. Conversely, we would expect that offenders who have not previously been in prison would have difficulty coping when they are imprisoned, because they have not learned the necessary adaptations. Thus, we should see a crossover: on the outside, coping would be inversely related to the amount of prison experience, but inside prison the relationship should be reversed. We shall examine this prediction when we turn to the data on subjects' lives in prison, in the following chapters. We can look at the relationships between previous prison experience, coping, and adaptation, and also, given our longitudinal design, at the changes in behavior over time for first-time inmates.

The simplest alternative explanation, and the one that we favor, assumes the primacy of coping ability. Everyday life is sometimes difficult for anyone. From the data we have presented here, we can conclude that offenders do not differ from anyone else in their problems. However, they do often cope poorly.

If we hypothesize that ineffective coping leads to maladaptive behavior, we can predict that poor coping, like that we saw among our subjects, will produce maladaptive behavior of one sort or another. The results will be seen in a variety of ways, not always undesirable: some people will show emotional problems, some may break under the stress and become psychotic or otherwise debilitated, but others may find effective help or simply devolve into eccentricity. If some individuals who cannot cope will become antisocial and violent, others may simply withdraw and find their own solitary fates, or resign themselves to lives of quiet desperation.

This coping–maladaptation hypothesis does not by itself deal specifically with the question of why some individuals commit violent or antisocial acts. It needs to be augmented by some mechanism that will predict which individuals will express their maladaptation in criminal behaviors. Given that we have shown a lifestyle pattern that is characteristic of offenders, we can hypothesize that people who cope poorly and also show patterns such as an unstructured impulsive lifestyle, dependence on frequent casual socialization, lack of planning or concern for the future, etc., will be those who are likely to commit criminal acts. Thus, the pattern of associated behaviors would function to channel the effects of inadequate coping ability into violent and antisocial actions.

We call this compound explanation the *coping–criminality* hypothesis. We would not claim that it can predict every form of criminal behavior, for there are certain classes of actions that are outside its scope. There are bound to be some well-adjusted criminals who act purely for material gain, those who are weak in the face of extraordinary temptations, or others who are under the spell of fanatical political or religious ideologies. Also, we would except those who commit offenses that are widely condoned by subgroups to which they belong, such as the use of cannabis, and those whose "criminality" is politically defined.

However, cases of these are atypical, at least in the Canadian experience: we saw no political prisoners and no religious zealots among our subjects, and at best only a very few who had links to "organized crime" (presumably to be distinguished from the disorganized crime characteristic of most offenders). Thus, the coping–criminality hypothesis is intended to deal with most examples of violent or habitual offenders seen in populations like those we examined.

This hypothesis is consistent with a number of findings already in the literature. For example, those guilty of repeated offenses show little consistency in the crimes for which they are convicted, and most men with long criminal records show convictions for a wide variety of offenses (Chaiken and Chaiken, 1982). Findings like this have been used to support notions of persistent dispositions toward criminality (the *bad seed* hypothesis), but they are also entirely consistent with the expectations of the coping explanation. The coping–criminality hypothesis will predict that an offense might occur, but it says that the details of the crime will depend largely on local circumstances of opportunity, experience, and elicitation.

Our hypothesis can also deal with many of the socioeconomic measures that have weak but reliable relationships with subsequent offending. We expect that these have their effects on the associated pattern of behaviors which channel maladaptation into criminal acts. For example, social class is linked with attitudes toward work and the use of time. Thus, a person of lower social class who suffers from the results of inadequate coping resources would be more likely to commit a criminal offense than another poorly adjusted individual with a different social background. Our hypothesis is consistent with the obtained linkage and also explains why it is weak. Similarly, we can understand why criminal careers so commonly begin in the early teen years for males: the lifestyle that predisposes men toward criminal offenses is in many ways very similar to that of a typical adolescent male social network, especially in such things as the pattern of numerous shallow social relationships and the importance of peer pressure.

There are also some predictions that can be tested with other parts of our data set. Poor coping outside of prison is associated with prior prison experience, and we might expect that this will also be true inside of prison. Thus, we can generate the paradoxical prediction that individuals with the least experience in prison may cope better with the conditions of imprisonment than those with extensive prison experience. This prediction is opposite to what might be expected if poor coping results from imprisonment.

In addition, we can test the prediction that poor coping leads to problems in adaptation using our data for life in prison. Since our design is longitudinal, we can use measures of coping and other behaviors at the first interview to see how well they predict adaptation over the subsequent period of a year or so. We would expect that poor coping will be associated with poor adaptation, regardless of prior experience in prison.

The coping–criminality hypothesis can also be applied in other areas. If particular factors lead to criminal acts, then we should be able not only to explain offenses postdictively, but also to predict recidivism among those who are released from prison. We can predict that the likelihood of a new offense will vary with the ability to cope with life outside of prison, as well as with the presence of the set of associated predisposing behaviors. Such a prediction is also testable.

In short, when we combine our results with our assumptions about the critical place of coping in adaptation, we arrive at a fairly comprehensive model for some of the principal factors in the causation of criminal behavior. The model makes some specific predictions about aspects of our data which we have not yet examined. Therefore, we shall turn to data on life inside prison before reconsidering the theoretical issues presented here.

6
The Impact of Imprisonment

The pattern of behavior that we saw for offenders on the outside was, of course, brought to an end by the process of arrest and imprisonment. In some cases the transition to the penitentiary was gradual, starting with a short stay after arrest and interrupted along the way by release on bail. In other cases the offender was not released at all between arrest and commitment to the penitentiary. However, in all cases the change was substantial, for the conditions in prison are very different than those in the outside world.

Therefore, we turn now to consideration of how subjects reacted to prison and how they were affected by the conditions they experienced. In this chapter we will look at conditions they faced at the beginning of their terms and how behavior was shaped by those conditions. In the next chapter we will consider in some detail the coping process inside prison and compare it to what we have seen for life on the outside. After that we will look at how things changed over the course of 16 months in prison, present the results of a survey of the effects of some particular factors, and finally consider how our measures can be used to predict subsequent adaptation in prison.

Although there have been many claims about generalized harmful effects of imprisonment, hard evidence is not easy to find. Previous arguments have been supported by citation of single cases or on intuitive grounds: if things are as unpleasant as they seem, they must be harmful. Therefore, we discounted much of the previous literature and set out as impartially as possible to see what were the effects of imprisonment on the general lot of prisoners. We shall first discuss how inmates' outside behavior patterns were disrupted by imprisonment, and then consider the evidence we have on their reactions.

Disruptions

The loose and unstructured lives led by many offenders on the outside are in sharp contrast to the regimentation of penitentiary. Fixed schedules are imposed, and variations from the behaviors expected at a particular time are followed by loss of rewards or privileges, or even by punishments. If coercion is not physical, it is nevertheless effective. Thus, for example, inmates are not actually physically turned out of bed if they do not rise at the expected time in the morning, but it is difficult to sleep when the lights are on at their brightest and the morning noises of a score of other men echo down long corridors and through the openings in cell doors. Meals are served at times convenient to the institution rather than to fit the hunger patterns of individuals. Of course, inmates have some freedom of choice in such things: they can eat what is served when it is served, or they can go hungry.

While the details vary across institutions, the general pattern is the same. To the outsider, what most distinguishes life in penal institutions from that elsewhere is its uniformity. Conditions in the institutions we surveyed are not inhumane, nor are they ususally imposed without some flexibility. For example, meals were usually of about the quality that one finds in institutions anywhere, including university dining halls. They provided a balanced diet of food in sufficient quantity to maintain good physical health. However, they were also uniform, bland, and predictable ("If I'm eating beef and macaroni, then today must be Thursday"). Inmates had few options for the inevitable days on which third-time leftovers were scheduled. At best, they could fill up on snack foods ordered once a week and paid for with their meager canteen funds.

Thus, for men used to living by the moment, the change appears substantial. Even when inmates can find a protective niche (Toch, 1977) they are still subject to the uniformity of routine, with little variation except that between weekdays and weekends.

When we look at the information we gathered on behavior patterns in prison, some differences from the outside become evident. First, we will consider what inmates did with their time within a day. As much as possible, the categories we used to group different sorts of activities were the same as those for life on the outside. The actual categories are shown in Table 6.1, with the mean daily times reported for activities in each. It can be seen that the total time specified was a bit less than for the outside, so we should emphasize the time in each category relative to others in the set.

The most significant change is probably in the category of work activities. In contrast to the outside, 96% of subjects were employed when we saw them, with the largest number, some 38%, in educational programs, and another 34% in training or trade programs. The average total for the work category of 31 hours weekly represents virtually full employment, as the institutional work week is nominally 32.5 hours and actually a bit shorter.

This is predictable from the demands made by the system. While basic physical necessities are provided almost unconditionally, additional items such as coffee between meals, shampoo, or postage stamps, must be

TABLE 6.1. Summary of average time usage inside prison at beginning of term (first interview).

Category	Mean daily hours
Sleep	7.1
Work, education or training	4.4
Socializing	3.7
Passive activity (TV, radio, recorded music)	2.9
Participatory activity (sports, hobbies)	1.7
Outside contact (letters, visits)	0.8
Group meetings	0.2
Other	1.8
Total	22.6

bought from funds earned within the institution. In addition, an inmate without a job assignment may be kept locked in his cell during working hours. Thus, we see how behavior is constrained to uniformity. Work was in effect a standard and required activity in prison; unlike what we saw for life on the outside, there was little variance in the time devote to it inside the penitentiary.

In contrast, the amounts of time spent in socializing and passive activities were somewhat reduced from what they were on the outside. The change in social activity is easily understood when one considers how great must be the effect of switching to a new environment. Most of our subjects' social networks were no longer available to them. Even for inmates who had served several previous terms, there were only a few familiar faces at the beginning of the term, given the rate of turnover in institutional populations. A substantial majority of respondents reported having had a greater number of friends outside of prison.

This does not mean that subjects were without social interactions. Indices of socialization are shown in Table 6.2, along with measures of a variety of other behaviors related to the use of time in prison. Given the previous importance of social activities in the lives of many subjects, one would expect that they would immediately begin to work on establishing new networks. Some began working on it as soon as they arrived.

The first thing I did was to find out who the solid (high status) guys were here, and then I introduced myself and tried to get in with them. It helps a lot to have the right friends.

It takes some time to identity potential friends and to establish friendships, and there was only a limited time for this to occur. About half of the sample said that at least a majority of their friendships in prison were with men they had met since the beginning of their current term, that is, in the previous month or so. Thus, for many subjects the pattern of casual and superficial friendships we saw for life on the outside was transported to

TABLE 6.2. Measures of specific behaviors related to use of time in prison (from first interview).

Variable	Percent	Mean
Time use categories		
Mean proportion of time in:		
Work		.30
Socializing		.23
Passive activity		.18
Sports and hobbies		.11
Visits and letters		.05
Group meetings		.02
Other things		.11
Employment		
Have a job in the institution	96.2	
Socialization		
Number of friends		1.7
Have no (0) friends	39.8	
Met majority of friends during term	46.3	
Pattern of socialization		
Stay on my own	42.9	
With a few friends	31.6	
In a larger group, or floating	21.8	
Mean percent of optional time spent in cell		29.9
Specified no (0) optional time in cell	30.3	
Spend majority of optional time in cell	20.5	
Outside contacts		
Number of visits received (month)		1.0
No (0) visits	38.6	
Number of visits desired (month)		2.2
No (0) visits desired	18.6	
Number of letters received (month)		3.4
No (0) letters	12.8	
Number of letters desired (month)		6.3
No (0) letters desired	8.4	
Frequency of reading or listening to news (wk)		7.8
Never read or listen to news	20.3	
Time framing		
Frequency of thoughts of future		
All of the time	22.3	
Most of the time	33.1	
Sometimes	20.8	
Rarely	17.3	
Never	6.2	
Frequency of thoughts of the past		
All of the time	9.2	
Most of the time	16.2	
Sometimes	34.6	
Rarely	32.3	
Never	7.7	

the new environment. If the rate of socialization was reduced from that on the outside, it was probably owing to the change in situations, and we would expect increasing socialization for the majority of inmates over the course of their time in prison.

At the same time, many inmates were very leery about opening themselves to possible entanglements from close friendships. In a crisis, friends are expected to provide support, and within prison this can often mean physical support in a fight. In consequence, many inmates (especially those with some previous experience in prison) preferred to limit the depth of their social alliances. When we asked them to characterize their preferred pattern of socialization from among a set of alternatives, 43% said that they preferred to be on their own, and another 32% chose "with a few close friends." Only 22% said that they wanted to be in larger social groups.

I just try to do my own time. I'm careful to say hello to everyone when I see them, and I spend some time with the guys on my block in the evenings. But they're not friends, more like neighbors, you have to get along with them. If you get involved with these guys you can end up in a jackpot and maybe wake up one morning with a knife in your back.

Still, few subjects chose not to engage at all in the prison social scene. During free hours when they had the choice, it was uncommon for subjects to stay in their cells by themselves. Only 20% stayed in their cells a majority of the time when they had the option, and even these men usually did so only to carry out some specific activity, e.g., studying or homework for their school programs. About half of the sample said that they stayed in their cell no more than 10% of the time when they had a choice. One reason for these low figures is the obvious physical unpleasantness of most cells, which made other places in the prison seem relatively more attractive.

Thus, in general, removal to prison disrupted subjects' social networks, but they were mostly able to rebuild the pattern on the inside, and in some ways the environment fostered these patterns. The penitentiary timetables are highly structured during usual working hours, but in the evenings and on weekends the inmates are mostly left with time to spend and a limited variety of diversions. Even though the opportunities for socialization are limited to a few hours daily, during those hours there are few alternatives. Inmates can either pass their time in the company of other inmates or do it alone in their cells. And there are not many choices for solitary cell activities, especially at the beginning of their terms. So, in a way, prison not only allows inmates to reestablish a social pattern like that on the outside, it almost forces it.

Some inmates respond by immersing themselves in the institutional social scene, giving themselves a perception of control by building social support and knowing about other inmates' positions. Others recognize that inmate social networks are bound up in the use of force and physical power that pervades social interactions in most institutions (Toch, 1969). In response to this, they are restrained and participate much less heartily, consciously trying to avoid entangling alliances. In the aggregate, the amount of socialization reported is fairly high, given the limited time available, but the majority of inmates try to keep the interactions superficial. To preserve their safety and their autonomy, they maintain some distance.

If we look at the other categories of time use in Table 6.1 we see that time in passive activities was lower than on the outside, but time in the category for sports and hobbies was increased. This is undoubtedly another consequence of the restricted choices available in prison. For example, although television facilities are available, they are situated in common rooms and the hours of access are restricted. Many inmates said that they rarely watched television in the institutions because they did not have their choice of programs, or because they would have to leave for the evening lockup before the end of the programs they wanted to watch. Communal facilities for records or tapes are lacking in most institutions, and although inmates can buy tape players as well as radios or televisions from their canteen funds, it takes some time to accumulate the necessary amount of money.

With the restrictions in diversionary activities, institutional recreational facilities become relatively attractive. Few inmates were involved in organized sports, but many regularly engaged in personal fitness programs. However, it is ironic that the most popular form of recreational activity is weight training, reinforcing the emphasis on physical power among inmates. Probably half of our subjects spent at least some time working out with weights. When we asked the reasons, we were almost always told explicitly that strong muscles were a good form of protection in the penitentiary. This may be part of the inmate mythology, for we suspect that well-developed muscles often provoke incidents, but there is no question that physical strength is a significant element in an inmate's status. In any case, it was a very popular activity and accounted for most of the time reported in our category for sports and hobbies.

The final change in time use from the outside is the result of a difference that is so obvious that it seems redundant to even point it out, but so profound that it probably outweighs all other differences. In contemporary prisons, inmates are not only removed from the free environment, they are also removed from their families and loved ones.

Although many men in our sample had spent only a limited amount of time with their families while on the outside, removal to prison provided a sharp break. At the time of the first interview, most inmates were in fact almost totally cut off from outside contact. Letters were infrequent, with an average of less than one a week. Visits from outsiders were also low, with a mean of only 1.0 monthly; 39% of the sample had no visits at all.

The infrequency of contacts was not by choice in most cases. When we asked about the desired number of letters and visits, we found that in each case subjects wanted much more than they had, and there were only a few prisoners who wanted no outside contacts at all. Most also tried to maintain other contacts with the outside, and received radio or television news broadcasts almost daily, at about the same frequency as on the outside.

As the penitentiary system operated at the time of this study, it took some time after a prisoner was transferred to an institution before his address was available for people wishing to write to him. At the other end, it might be a few weeks before an inmate could buy writing materials and stamps to send mail out. As for visits, it usually took a month or two for lists of likely visitors to be compiled and approved. In the meantime, inmates were on their own, without the possibility of direct contact with the outside world, with the occasional exception of communication with someone involved with the determination of their legal status, e.g., lawyers or family caseworkers. It made it easy to understand why they were so willing to talk with us.

Thus, from our survey of time usage in prison, we can see many of the special conditions to which inmates are subject, and also some of the ways those conditions affect behavior. We see how the requirement of a work assignment produces a uniform amount of time to be spent on the job, at the cost of time in other activities. On the other hand, we also see how the separation from family on the outside leaves a real gap in many inmates' lives—and not just a gap in their time schedules.

On the outside, most inmates had been poor in dealing with choices or in structuring their lives. In prison they do not have these difficulties, for few areas in their lives allow alternatives of their own devising, and many important areas allow no choices at all. They must spend the specified times working in one of the limited selection of available employments, while at other specified times they may find entertainments in the allocated places from among the choices they are allowed. The restrictions on time are accompanied by restrictions on physical movement. Inmates are always limited as to the places where they are allowed to be at any given time, and sometimes they have no choice at all; for example, they are required to be in their cells about half of their total time. Of course, all of this is done while dressed in the clothing provided . . . etcetera, etcetera.

When we add together the large changes, and consider all of the small ways they can manifest themselves, we can see how much change the fact of imprisonment can impose on an individual's life. We do not pretend or intend to provide here an exhaustive and complete description of the special conditions of imprisonment. There are many other aspects that we have omitted, but they have been described in other places. However, we can see how the prison environment imposes a strong set of constraints operating at every minute of inmates' lives, with the effect of homogenizing their lives in many ways.

We believe that the system is not deliberately rigid, but it is certainly bureaucratic. If an inmate needed a special pair of shoes they were usually provided, but it might take months. Another inmate might desire a special diet; again, he could usually get it if he had a good medical or religious reason, but not before the request had been through a pyramid of approvals, and even then he might still have to sweet talk the kitchen workers into actually providing what he wanted. In the quiet contrast of our own institutional settings, we were haunted by the specter of our lives as they might be if run by the Post Office. Sometimes it seemed a fit analogy.

Negative Effects

With the disruption in customary behavior caused by imprisonment, and also the restrictions, deprivations, and constraints imposed, we would expect some deleterious reactions. Human beings are extraordinarily adaptable, but change does not occur without some cost. There were certainly strong indications of strain among our subjects when we interviewed them at the beginnings of their sentences, apparent in some of the measures of Table 6.3.

Certainly they were not happy with the conditions they faced. When asked to rate their lives on a scale from 0 to 100, the mean rating was only about 35, and only 20% gave ratings above 50. When asked to list positive aspects of their imprisonment, over one-third could find nothing at all, and another 21% mentioned only educational and training opportunities.

When we look at measures of emotional state, a number of indications of disturbance can be seen. For example, although the mean time spent sleeping was virtually the same as that reported for outside of prison, there were many reports of sleeping problems. Just under half had a sleep problem at the first interview, more than twice the number who reported difficulties on the outside. In the great majority of cases, the problem was some difficulty in falling asleep, typically because of arousing or troubling thoughts. This is evidence of at least a temporary increase in emotional discomfort.

More serious indications can be seen in our measures of depression and anxiety. We had used the Beck Depression Inventory to assess overall mood state, since it is the most widely used measure of its kind. The mean score for the entire sample was 13.0, near the top of the "mildly depressed" range and close to the level considered diagnostic of clinical depression for an individual. What is more disturbing is that 29% of subjects had scores in the "moderately depressed" range and a further 8% had scores classed as "severely depressed." The incidence of scores in the latter category was about 8 times that in the general population, and for the former category it was about 5 times the usual rate. Although there was a (small and statistically nonsignificant) tendency for more of the long-term

TABLE 6.3. Measures of emotional state and motivations to change in prison (from first interview).

Variable	Percent	Mean
General appraisals		
General rating of quality of life (0–100)		35.4
Rated quality of life at 50 or below	80.0	
Specified "No (0) positive things here"	35.9	
Expectations		
Have appeals of sentence or conviction	42.1	
Estimated chance of appeal success (0–100)		62.3
Estimated chance of earliest parole (0–100)		59.9
Emotions		
Self-reported sleeping problems	48.1	
Frequency of emotion (week, self-report):		
Depression		3.0
Anger		2.0
Anxiety		2.8
Guilt feelings		1.5
Boredom		4.1
Reported no (0)		
Depression	30.1	
Anger	40.6	
Anxiety	35.1	
Guilt feelings	63.6	
Boredom	35.3	
Score on Beck Depression Inventory		13.0
Score on Spielberger State Anxiety Inventory		46.8
Score on Hopelessness Scale		4.7
Score on Self-esteem Scale		6.2
Frequency of missing people from outside		
All of the time	39.2	
Most of the time	36.8	
Sometimes	14.4	
Rarely	3.2	
Never	6.4	
Planning		
Reported general plan for doing time	83.5	
Reported having goal for term	80.5	
Specified that goal is education or training	74.8	
Specified that goal is behavior change	13.6	
In educational or vocational training programs	69.2	
Reported choosing job for self-improvement	60.2	
Planned time (vs living day-by-day)	21.0	
Attempts to control thoughts		
Try to think about things	37.3	
Try not to think about things	27.3	
Just let thoughts happen	35.5	
Cognitions		
Mean Internal-External Scale (external)		48.2
Mean Attitudes Toward Criminal Justice System		72.2
Self-categorizations		
Doing time (avoid trouble, get out soon)	39.4	
Gleaning (better myself, profit from the time)	51.5	
Jailing (forget the outside, have a good time)	9.1	

inmates to appear several depressed, indications of depression seemed to be spread across all subgroups, regardless of previous experience or other background factors.

Confirmation of a problem comes from the scores on the Hopelessness Scale, where one-third of subjects had scores of 6 or higher. Although diagnostic categories on this scale have not been defined as they have for the Beck, scores as high as we found are undeniable indications of depression, and even possible suicidal tendencies.

We cannot say from these numbers that a large proportion of our sample was clinically depressed, for the diagnosis of depression involves more than can be seen on any simple self-report assessment. However, we can say that a high proportion of those individuals would ordinarily be found to be in need of treatment, and many would be hospitalized. Given the link between depression and a variety of undesirable or even calamitous outcomes, from illness to suicide, we conclude that a real problem is evident.

A similar result was obtained with our measure of anxiety, the Spielberger State Anxiety Index. The original standardization of this test (Spielberger, Gorsuch, and Lushene, 1970) included means for several groups, one of which was a group of prison inmates with a mean of 46.0. Our figure (46.8) is obviously in agreement with this standardization value. However, it should be noted that the mean score for the inmate group reported by Spielberger et al. was much higher than that for a group of university students (36.3) and close to that for a group of psychiatric patients diagnosed as suffering from anxiety reactions (49.0).

Our obtained mean value thus indicates that a substantial number of our subjects had elevated anxiety levels. In fact, 41% had scores above the mean for the anxiety reaction patients. On this evidence we conclude that a clinical anxiety problem existed initially among the inmates in this study, as well as a similar pattern of depression. Since depression and anxiety often occur together in individuals, it is not surprising that they were both apparent in our group of subjects.

These data show that emotional disruption is clearly a problem among inmates beginning a new term. They also suggest the need for more psychological treatment than is usually available at present. We expect that the lives of both inmates and correctional staff would be easier if the emotional states of new inmates were routinely and carefully assessed at the time of admission, and if those who appeared to need it were offered treatment.

While the evidence for emotional disturbance is undeniable, we should make it clear that we cannot say for certain that it was an effect of imprisonment. We had not measured emotional states in our subjects before they were arrested or imprisoned, and it is possible that the disturbances we saw were chronic and/or long-term and that they existed before imprisonment. However, we think this unlikely because the sort of disturbed emotional states we saw are usually reactive, i.e., they occur in response to some strong situational determinants. Arrest, conviction, and imprisonment were the only major evens that subjects had in common that might have provoked major emotional upsets, so we conclude somewhat cautiously that these events were the cause of the upsets. If we are correct, we would expect that the disturbance would lessen after subjects had more time to acclimate to the conditions of imprisonment. In chapter 8, we will look at the evidence for such changes.

While we are surveying emotional states after arrival in prison, one other type of evidence is perhaps relevant. In addition to the standardized tests, we also asked subjects how often they experienced each of a variety of emotional states. Results for depression and anxiety were consistent with the measures already presented. However, the emotions we surveyed included feelings of both anger and guilt, states not otherwise measured. The frequency of anger was lower than expected, with episodes on an average of 2.0 days per week, clearly less than the values for both depression and anxiety, and also about 20% less than frequencies of anger reported by subjects for life outside of prison.

The results for guilt were also quite interesting. About 64% of the sample reported that they never felt such a state—even though most freely admitted they had actually committed the crimes for which they were convicted. Moreover, the frequency of guilt feelings reported for life in prison was about a third less than that for life on the outside previous to imprisonment. When we asked some of those who did report guilt feelings to give some details of their occurrence, they said that the feelings were attached to recall of their crimes; as the memories became less frequent with the passage of time, the feelings were evoked less frequently. Thus, inmates may often undergo many dysphoric emotions, but rarely does imprisonment induce in them much guilt or remorse.

Positive Effects

As we have seen, the contrast between conditions in the outside world and the environment in prison leads to considerable emotional distress in many inmates. But the disruption of old patterns, and/or the consequent dysphoria, also seemed to have some effects that could be beneficial. As a result, the majority of inmates seemed amenable to change at the beginning of their terms. This may be seen in some of the measures in the bottom part of Table 6.3.

Subjects' attempts to change and improve themselves can be seen in examining their plans and objectives for their terms. Eighty percent said that they had a goal to accomplish during the term, with the great majority of these specifying either education or job training, and half of the remainder specifying ways of changing or reforming their behavior to prevent a return to prison. Most also said they had chosen their job or training program with self-improvement as the primary benefit in mind.

To get an idea of subjects' overall approach to their time in prison, we asked them to assign themselves to one of three categories of inmates described by Irwin (1970). A clear majority identified themselves with the description of "gleaners," i.e., those who work to use the prison experience for self-improvement and to better themselves. In comparison, 39% said that they were trying to avoid trouble and get out as soon as possible ("doing time") and only 9% said that they tried to forget the outside and have as good a time as possible in their institutions ("jailing").

So, if most inmates found prison decidedly unpleasant or even painful, a great many of them wanted to try to profit from the experience. Some even said that they were grateful that they had been caught, because they had been in intolerable situations on the outside from which they could not extricate themselves.

You know, I really hate this place, but it's probably all for the best. I was in over my head out there, just destroying myself with drinking, and I couldn't stop. I was getting kind of desperate. And then they caught me and I end up in this miserable place, but it's my own fault. I don't know what kind of terrible things I might have done if they didn't stop me when they did. Sometimes, I thank God that I got caught and stopped and got another chance to straighten myself out. I wish they had got me sooner.

It was our impression that subjects were split into three groups. One group, consisting mostly of very experienced criminals with records of serious violence, seemed to fit immediately into the prison routine. Like Irwin's (1970) description of inmates "doing time," they accepted the institutional regime with little apparent resentment, and wanted only to get through their time with the least possible trouble. Many had not been free for very long, and they returned to the routine as most of us do after an extended holiday (cf., Manocchio and Dunn, 1970). We would judge that 20–25% of subjects fit into this classification.

At the other extreme were subjects who took a uniformly optimistic view of their terms. Like the inmate quoted above, they were grateful that they had been apprehended and fully expected that their lives would be changed. For example, 11% said that prison benefited them because it broke the cycle of undesirable behavior, and 13% rated the quality of their lives in prison at 60 or above (on our 100-point scale). These subjects were not critical of the conditions they found in prison, deciding in a Panglossian way that they were all for the best. Three or four had become religious converts, although most put their faith in more secular means of salvation such as Alcoholics Anonymous or the Correctional Service of Canada.

Together, these two groups probably accounted for no more than one-third of the sample, for most fell into a middle category with mixed characteristics. Paradoxically, the majority of subjects were resentful, critical, and likely bitter about their experiences with the penal system, but also optimistic about the future, especially their chances for reform and success after their release. We were struck by the number of subjects who spontaneously specified that they were "not like those other guys": they shared the public image of convicts as permanent criminals, but they did not see themselves as fitting the mold. They felt that their crimes had been aberrations (though their record sheets were sometimes extensive) and fully expected that they could and would change.

Thus, we believe that there is good evidence that a real opportunity for changing subjects' behavior existed at the beginning of their terms. However, it seemed unlikely to us that real changes would occur for many, for good intentions and vague expectations do not provide the means for significant changes in behavior. Although 91% said that they had plans for the future, the great majority were vague, unclear, or unrealistic.

My girlfriend's father is out West. When I get out, we'll go there and I can get a job. Then we'll get married and settle down, I always wanted to do that. (What sort of job?) Well, I don't know yet, I got three years to decide.

Even with their hopes and plans for the future, most subjects actually thought about it infrequently, as can be seen in some of the results in Table 6.2. On our 5-point scale, the mean value was 2.5, a little better than on the outside but still not very much if one is planning a future life. Even planning of time in the immediate future was no better than it had been on the outside, and 79% still lived day by day, rather than planning.

No, I don't plan my time. Do I live day by day? No, a day's a long time in here, too much to think about. I just let things happen. I guess you'd say I live minute by minute.

Thus, old habits and patterns regarding planning and the use of time seemed well established. While imprisonment changed a great deal in subjects' external environment, it had little direct impact on most of their ways of dealing with the world. We can see the same thing in other areas of behavior, e.g., social interactions: although the cast of characters was changed, the pattern of loose interactions with an extended network of people remained. And when we consider coping in the next chapter, we will see parallel results. In many ways, imprisonment reinforces the behaviors that inmates bring to prison.

One may ask why this would be so. One answer is that prisons are in some way responsible for creating the pattern. Unfortunately, we have no evidence of any such process, and we have several findings that argue against it, as will be more apparent later. Alternatively, it may be argued that prison policies have been shaped historically by inmate behavior, rather than the reverse. When conditions match the propensities of inmates, then authorities will find that the management of institutions is easier and problems are fewer. Thus, prisons allow inmates to recreate on the inside some of the pattern of their lives on the outside, and they therefore allow those behaviors to be perpetuated and even reinforced.

As a result, we would expect that little would be different when inmates are ultimately released from prison. If they remain essentially unchanged, they will fall back into the pattern that led most of them into the acts for which they were imprisoned. We would expect that without significant behavioral change their vague and optimistic hopes for the future would soon be forgotten. Only in rare cases was there available the opportunity for effective help in changing behavior, such as relevant treatment programs. Hopes without means are of little consequence. In the end, we felt we had begun to see why prisons do not work in reforming criminals. They constrain the body, but they leave unaffected a great deal of inmates' behavior and ways of thinking. Considering that what lands men in prison is the way they think and behave, this is illogical.

It is also very unfortunate. An essential requisite for behavioral change is a strong and reliable motivation. The impact of the beginning of a term in penitentiary was considerable for the majority of inmates, and could provide the necessary motivation. Misery is one of the best motivators, and the evidence in this chapter indicates that emotional distress was strikingly high at the first interview. In addition, the conditions we surveyed at the beginning of this chapter are sufficient to break up many old patterns, at least temporarily, to allow room for new ways of acting. Thus, we see the shock of imprisonment opening a window of opportunity. However, we expect that the window will close with the passage of time, unless the winds of change blow through it.

7
Coping in Prison

In the previous chapter, we considered some of the restrictions imposed by imprisonment, and the consequences for inmates' behavior and emotions. However, we have not yet shown how aspects of the general experience are translated into particular and personal problems experienced by inmates, nor have we considered specific and individual ways of reacting to circumstances in prison. Therefore, we turn now to consideration of the problems seen by subjects within prison and the ways they dealt with those problems, just as we looked before at coping on the outside.

Problems in Prison

We assessed the problems experienced by inmates in prison as we had done for life on the outside. The prompts used in the inquiry were based on preliminary interviews and previous experience with prisoners, so they were quite different from those for the outside, but the procedures for producing individual lists of problems were the same.

Subjects found it easy to specify problems in prison life. None failed to supply at least two items, and the mean number of problems was 20% higher than on the list for life outside of prison. This had been expected, but it does not necessarily mean that the prison environment was really more stressful, for it might reflect only the greater currency and recency of life in the penitentiary. Memory tends to wipe away past emotional distress selectively, while present trifles are sometimes magnified by their immediacy. For example, we saw instances when an inmate was subjected to an unusually thorough search on the way to the interview room, and then listed harassment from guards as one of his most important problems, although this complaint was otherwise relatively infrequent.

In any case, the problems were almost all current, chronic, and specific to the situation in prison. This may be seen from the list of the most common problems shown in Table 7.1. As with the outside problems, the categories in this list were generated after inspection of the problems specified in the interviews.

TABLE 7.1. Common problem categories inside prison at beginning of term (first interview).

Category	Frequency	Percent
1. Missing family or friends	107	82
2. Missing freedom	57	44
3. Missing specific object or activity	45	35
4. Conflicts with other inmates	41	32
5. Regrets or troubling thoughts about past	40	31
6. Concern re future, esp. life after release	40	31
7. Boredom	33	25
8. Cell conditions (privacy, noise, etc.)	23	18
9. Medical services	19	15
10. Lack of staff support or help	18	14
11. Concern about personal safety	16	12
12. Lack of desired programs or facilities	14	11

The great majority of subjects were troubled by the separation from loved ones on the outside, and for most of them the problem of missing someone ranked near the top of their lists. This category clearly dominates the choices. Problems with the loss of freedom because of imprisonment comprised the second most frequent category, but this was listed by only about half the number of subjects who had reported missing people. From here down, there was still more of a dropoff in frequency. Among the other 10 categories, 8 are specific to conditions inside the institutions.

While the list contains no surprises, it illustrates how imprisonment presents a variety of hassles and restrictions that dominate the concerns of inmates. After the drama of arrest and trial, life settles into a mundane level where the uniformity is punctuated by petty confrontations, minor deprivations, and bureaucratic restrictions. The ever-present absence of loved ones presents itself often and unpredictably, in small ways as well as large.

After a few weeks in prison, inmates had begun to take many of its restrictions for granted. What reminded them of their loss of freedom and choice was not so much the larger differences from life on the outside, but the little things. When we asked them what they missed most from the outside, they rarely mentioned major things (except people) but rather the small remembered pleasures of which they were deprived. In the winter they would tell us how they missed walking through the snow, and in the summer we heard about missing the chance to lie in the sun. Sometimes the answers were surprising.

This will sound stupid, but what I really miss most is ketchup. Sometimes I think that if I had my own bottle of ketchup to put on my food whenever I wanted, I could be happy here. (Supplies of ketchup were restricted because it could be used for making alcohol.)

We are sure that such answers were not literally correct, but they probably did honestly express concerns of the moment. In the constant flux of daily life, major situations often manifest themselves for us in trifles, and it is often these that seem to make the most difference to us. As marriages founder on unwashed dishes, or kingdoms fail for want of a nail, so do prisoners often become depressed because of the absence of ketchup on the breakfast table or the impossibility of getting a favorite brand of shampoo. Thus, we can see how routine diverts people from other concerns: more subjects were concerned with the absence of some object from the outside (e.g., their cars or clothing) than with planning their futures, and boredom was far more frequent than fears for their personal safety.

On one hand, we can see the success of efforts to make the Canadian prison system more humane over the last decade, for on the whole inmates seemed to feel that basic necessities were adequately provided for. On the other hand, we can also see the limits to the usefulness of such improvement programs, for many of the problems listed are inherent in the nature of imprisonment, or are unavoidable with the physical arrangements conventional in contemporary penitentiaries.

The types of problems expressed by our sample of Canadian inmates are quite similar to those expressed by British and American prisoners in previous studies (Richards, 1978; Flanagan, 1980). Our list shows how the fact of imprisonment dominates prisoners' lives. Not only does it constrain their behaviors, as we saw in the last chapter, but it determines also their choice of problems. As prison life is more uniform and predictable than that on the outside, so are the problems that inmates experience less varied. The prison experience is sufficiently powerful that it nullifies much of the variance among inmates, and they come to resemble each other much more than before imprisonment.

We looked at whether the choice of problems on an inmate's list was related to other important variables, and found no apparent relationships. For example, long-term subjects were not significantly more likely to report any given problem than short-term subjects, and inmates who had never before been in prison seemed to have the same sorts of problems as those with long histories of previous imprisonment. Moreover, there were no great differences across the different institutions in which subjects were kept. Again, we must say that the nature of imprisonment enforces a uniformity that overshadows other differences.

Coping in Prison: Categories

Given the problems summarized in Table 7.1, and the restrictions and conditions discussed in the previous chapter, we can now consider how subjects actually responded to specific situations in prison.

We gathered data in the interview in the same way as for data on coping

TABLE 7.2. Coping modes used on the outside previous to current term and at beginning of term in prison (first interview).

Category	Percentage of Subjects Using	
	Outside	Inside
None (giving up)	2	8
Reactive Problem-oriented	100	96
Avoidance	46	50
Escape	30	61
Palliative	52	62
Social Support	32	21
Anticipatory Problem-oriented	13	16
Reinterpretive (Re-evaluation)	7	23
Reinterpretive (Self-control)	10	32
Substitution	12	18
Drug-taking	64	3

with problems on the outside, and then we classified and analysed them in the same manner. The results show the continuation of many of the ways of responding we had seen with problems outside of prison, and for the most part subjects were not any better in dealing with their problems in prison than they had been on the outside. However, in some ways their responses were relatively more effective in dealing with the conditions in prison than on the outside. At the same time, there were also some differences in coping that followed from the restraints of imprisonment. All of this will be elaborated in the next few pages.

We can compare coping in prison with that on the outside by first examining the use of our categories of coping responses. Table 7.2 compares initial frequencies for behavior in prison with the values for behavior on the outside shown earlier in chapter 5.

We can see first that there was little change in either of the problem-oriented. The most common way of dealing with problems was still the direct low-level sort of response classified as Reactive Problem-oriented. For example, when the problem was missing someone on the outside, the most frequent response was to write a letter. Similarly, most inmates reported that when they were bored they would "go find something to do." In the circumstances, these are effective actions, probably more so than actions classified in the same category for behavior on the outside. However, they are also limited in their effectiveness, and would have little permanent effect on the chronic long-term problems they typically addressed.

If we look at responses in the Anticipatory Problem-oriented class, we can see that here also there was little change from the outside. Thus, inmates were still dealing with their problems in direct but unsystematic ways, without much evidence of organized or planned attack. As exceptions, there were some examples of good problem analysis and concerted action for long-term benefit. Consider the following:

I really miss my wife and children. I feel cut off from them, and can't communicate. (Specifically?) Well, once I didn't get a letter for nearly two weeks, and I was convinced something terrible happened to one of the kids, like they were dying from some sickness, and my wife didn't want to tell me. (What do you do about it?) Whenever I think about them and feel lonely I take out my wife's letters and read them over, and then I write a letter. For a while that's all I did, but then I decided I could be doing the same thing every night for the next 5 years, so I figured I had to make a plan to get out of here. I talked to (classification officer) and asked about transfers to minimum and he said that it would take probably a year even if I didn't get into trouble. So I wake up every day and tell myself "keep cool, you got to get out of here." I want to convince them that I'm a good inmate, then they'll help me to get to a minimum and day parole. I changed my job to training in the machine shop even though I don't like it, to show them how I'm serious, and I go to all the group meetings I can. And then when I feel lonely I tell myself "Not too long now, just keep cool."

However, responses like this were infrequent, with only one out of six subjects showing any evidence of such planning, even with the resolve to better themselves that we have already discussed. Although prison presents to offenders much time for contemplation, it does not lead them to plan or organize their behavior any better than before.

If we except problem-oriented responses, we can see from the table that overall the most frequently used response categories are those we have considered as lower-level coping behaviors. This is again similar to responses to outside problems, except that there were some differences in individual categories.

The largest change was for Escape responses, which was used by about twice as many inmates as on the outside. In a way this is paradoxical, because one does not think of a prison as a place where problems can be escaped. There are strong limitations on where an inmate can go, and also on the range of possible activities that he can use for shifting his attention.

Still, escape—at least as we have defined it—was a very frequent way of dealing with problems. Probably this was because the category included responses that did not involve physical removal from a situation, especially those in which the escape was from troubling thoughts or images.

Escape of this sort is particularly suited to the nature of the problems reported. The three most frequent problems all involved deprivations, defined in terms of features of a normal environment that were missing in prison. In addition, problems five and six were specifically defined as the occurrence of troubling thoughts. Instances when problems were felt were often—if not typically—triggered by some event in the prison. For example, one subject said that he would awake every morning in a good mood, and try to pretend that he was in a cheap hotel while on a foreign holiday; this worked until he needed to use the toilet and could not fail to notice the missing seat, which brought home to him the restrictions under which he was living, destroyed his consoling stratagem, and often made him feel depressed for hours. In the same way, many things can act as the taste of madeleine that reminds the prisoner of the things he cannot have.

Once an inmate was reminded of his problem, the difficulties troubling him were prominently in his thoughts. This is not unusual, for the same thing happens for all of us with our problems on the outside. However, when such troubling thoughts appeared in prison, inmates most often dealt with them by finding ways of terminating them.

Usually, I think about some of the good times we had. That makes me feel good but then it makes me sad, so I try to take my mind off it. Sometimes the thoughts come back in four seconds, but I do something else to not think about it, anything else that keeps my head busy.

A very common strategy was to divert attention with physical action.

When it gets bad I go to the gym and do some weights. Sometimes I work out until I'm so tired my mind just turns off.

The category of coping responses most similar to Escape is Avoidance. Although there is not much difference between Escape and Avoidance, the latter requires a bit of forethought, or at least earlier action, in order to forestall an event or thought before it occurs. Responses in this category were quite common in prison, almost as frequent as Escape.

It (thinking of his family) always gets me down, so I just avoid thinking of them. I put the letters out of sight so they don't remind me, and I keep busy so it doesn't creep into my head.

The number of subjects classified as using responses in the Avoidance category did not increase in prison, as did Escape. This may have been because Avoidance was already so common on the outside. However, there were some differences between the responses outside and those in prison. On the outside, responses in this category were primarily physical avoidance of a troubling place or situation. On the inside, as we have already discussed, physical avoidance was difficult. Also, problems in prison more often involved troubling thoughts. Even with planning and deliberate strategy, the ability to control thoughts from within is a rather difficult skill that most inmates lack.

While responses in the Escape and Avoidance categories were the most common ways of coping, they were rarely used exclusively. Once thoughts had been dealt with, subjects had a variety of ways to alleviate the consequent unpleasant feelings. This included talking with other inmates for information, solace, or just diversion, all included under the category of Social Support. As one might expect, this was less frequent than on the outside, because of the disruption of old relationships that we have already discussed.

However, there was a lot of variety in the things subjects reported they did to improve their mood, i.e., Palliative responses. When they felt keenly the absence of certain people, memories or imagination were often very helpful.

When I miss my wife, I look at her pictures. Sometimes I think of some of our good times. Or I think about something funny that happened to us, and I laugh, it helps when you laugh.

I miss sex and also female companionship. When I feel down about it, I read a letter or write one. If I don't have a new letter I read old ones, they're still a pick-me-up and I feel better until I get a new one. I also have this thing with my wife, twice a week we both pretend we're together, like transcending. I close my eyes and talk to her, and if I know she's doing the same thing it's almost like we're really together.

Another very common palliative was the thought of a successful appeal that would put an end to the discomforts of prison. Despite the actual rarity of successful appeals, those who were appealing (42%) estimated their chances of success on the average as better than even.

For many subjects, belief in the magical deliverance of an appeal was an important way of coping. In its promise that the present situation was temporary, it helped them to live through what might otherwise have been intolerable. This was particularly true in the case of some subjects with 15- or 25-year minimum terms. Even though most probably knew objectively that the chances of their appeal's being successful were slim, its existence was an important palliative to them.

I have two terms to serve: the first is from now until my appeal is over, and the second is the rest of the 25 years if I lose my case.

Similarly, there were also unrealistic expectations about the chances of early release. The average estimate of the chance of release at the earliest possible date (one-third of the sentence with the granting of parole, except in the case of life terms with specified minimum times) was 60%, very unrealistic if one considers the low proportion of applications approved by the parole board. The median inmate said that he expected to serve only 37% of his sentence. Again, subjects frequently consoled themselves with thoughts of deliverance, and if their expectations were incorrect they may nevertheless have been appropriate simply for their palliative value.

In addition, a variety of other diversionary activities were sometimes used as palliatives. Some subjects reported listening to sad music on the radio, others avoided the sad songs and turned to music with strong driving rhythms. Some found solace in reading, others avoided it because it allowed their thoughts to wander. Some wanted to do hobbycraft because of the rewards of creating, others gambled for the excitement. Some even worked on schemes of escape from prison that they never really planned to implement. Palliative actions were distinguished by their individuality and their variety.

Thus, in general subjects showed a dependence on low-level types of coping responses in prison, much as they had done on the outside. If the frequency of Escape responses was increased some, and Social Support decreased, the changes are understandable in terms of the constraints of imprisonment. As always, the details of coping were shaped by the situation. However, it seems that imprisonment made no substantial difference in the underlying pattern of reactive and low-level reponding. Subjects who entered prison with deficient skills were not immediately changed.

However, there were some changes in overall responding that did appear. The most profound difference was in a way also trivial, as it too was forced by the nature of imprisonment: drug-taking was almost abolished. There is currently some concern that alcohol and other drugs are easily available in prison, and a few subjects did report current use even though we had not asked for specific information about drugs in prison. Nevertheless, compared to the rates of consumption on the outside, drug use was vastly reduced after imprisonment.

From one perspective this is certainly fortunate, as the level of alcohol use reported for the outside was sufficient to produce major organic damage if continued over time; at the least, interruption by a period for recovery in prison would have been beneficial to many subjects. On the other hand, the loss of drugs as a way of avoiding problems ought to have forced inmates to find some new ways of coping. We can see some of the adjustment in the increased rate of Escape responses, but there is no evidence that the restriction of drug usage led to any real improvement in coping ability.

Another change, which may actually indicate some changes in coping behavior, was a substantial increase in the number of subjects using Reinterpretive or cognitive types of coping.

I can't change it in here. Most of the time I tell myself to accept this situation, in only 4 more months I can start applying for parole.

I tell myself that God must have a purpose for putting me here; and then I look around at other inmates here, and I can see that I'm lucky by comparison.

Our two categories for this sort of response are very similar, both requiring some abstract representation of the problem and then a reduction of its stressful properties by thoughts or an inner dialogue (what many contemporary cognitive therapists call "self talk"). As such, they probably represent a higher level of coping than the other types commonly used by inmates. Subjects had rarely reported these types of responses in dealing with problems outside of prison, and the appearance of one or the other in about a third of our subjects was unexpected.

We have no convincing explanation for the appearance of cognitive strategies in prison. In part they probably reflect the great persistence of problems in prison. Some of the chronic problems experienced by inmates are inescapable consequences of placement in a prison. Once they begin to trouble someone, they will not likely disappear, although they might be overshadowed by other problems that arise. If an inmate is troubled by missing his family at the beginning of his term, it will be some time before he forgets them, and in the meantime he will be reminded frequently of his deprivations. Given that problems in prison are largely in the nature of thoughts, if the ways they are ordinarily handled are not adequate to prevent some discomfort, then we might expect that attempts to find some alternatives would often be cognitive in nature.

However, as we stressed earlier, the type of responses one makes is not so important as their quality. Even if inmates had begun to use cognitive strategies, there is no reason to think that they used them well, or that the result was any more effective than their previous attempts at coping. Still, the use of new types of responses shows the capacity for improvement, something that good training programs could make use of (Ross and Fabiano, 1985).

The Quality of Coping in Prison

In summary, we can say that there were only minor differences in the types of responses that we saw for problems in prison from those used on the outside. Therefore, we expected that ratings of the effectiveness of responses would be similar to the poor levels for the outside. However, the rated levels of efficacy for coping responses within prison were somewhat higher than those for the outside. For example, the mean score on the benefits scale was 2.92, very close to a mediocre level and clearly higher than the value for coping on the outside. We stratified scores into three groups: scores of 2.5 or lower were considered as poor; the mediocre range was from 2.5 to 3.5; and values above 3.5 were classified as good. Using these criteria, 45% of the sample had scores in the poor range on the outside, but only 17% on the inside. Only 12% qualified as good copers on the outside, but 38% on the inside.

One can see an even more impressive change in the ratings of risk, that is, scores for responses that would likely make things worse. While 70% of inmates had ratings indicating that their responses to at least one outside problem carried some risk, for prison problems the figure was only 14%.

Since the overall Efficacy score was defined as the product of benefits and risks, we would expect higher ratings for coping behavior inside prison than outside. The mean value was 11.6 for the inside as compared to 8.0 for the outside, a statistically significant difference ($t = 11.5, p < .001$).

This might seem paradoxical, given that there was not a lot of difference in the types of coping responses used in the two environments. However, it was certainly not an artifact of the rating procedures, for the ratings were all done by the same individuals, and the order of rating was randomized. Rather, the differences in ratings emphasize some of the differences between life in prison and that on the outside.

Within the penitentiary, the range of possible actions available to a person is very limited compared to what is possible outside. As we have seen, most of the problems that inmates see as important within prison are the results of either specific institutional conditions or of the constraints imposed by the fact of imprisonment itself. In the same way, the actions available to inmates are also constrained: they are not only in conformity with institutional requirements, but they are more uniform, with less variance.

One aspect of this is shown in the risk ratings. As the behaviors from which inmates may choose are constrained, many of the ineffective, diversionary, or destructive actions they might take on the outside are precluded. Looking at their coping responses inside of prison, it is clear that many of the damaging responses available on the outside (e.g., get drunk until I can't remember the problem, try to intimidate people who don't give me what I want, hit the wife who argues with me) are either very difficult or else very dangerous inside the penitentiary.

However, imprisonment does more than simply prevent counterproductive coping responses. While an inmate can still avoid a problem, or deal with it ineffectively, it is more difficult to avoid facing it in some fashion. An inmate's problems in prison are almost inevitably part of his daily life and routine, and they are evoked or encountered regularly, because the institutional world is so confined and restricted. In effect, prison creates the problems, defines the possible responses to those problems, and then requires the inmate to choose from among the available options.

We must remember that many of the most serious problems experienced by prisoners are insoluble. The responses that our subjects had mastered were those of evasion and low-level temporary management; with insoluble problems these were often relatively effective. In a way, the restrictions of imprisonment set up conditions in which the ways offenders cope are relatively appropriate, and the average ratings of effectiveness are bound to be higher than those for life under less constrained conditions. In addition, imprisonment prevents most of the inappropriate and damaging actions so commonly used by offenders on the outside.

Thus, the constraints of imprisonment extend not only to physical confinement and the enforcement of rules, but they also work on almost all aspects of the coping process. The same restrictions that create many problems work paradoxically to make inmates deal relatively more effectively with those problems. One might say that they are not free to cope so badly in prison as they did on the outside.

In addition, inmates often provide some help for each other in dealing with prison conditions. Given that their problems in prison are often very similar, it is not surprising that they have a shared culture on coping. We could see this when we asked about their general plans for getting through their terms: "Do your own time" was usually the predictable answer. Sometimes the tutoring of other inmates was probably an impediment to solving problems, for example when it advised inmates that staff members could never be trusted. However, on the whole it was certainly a useful resource for most inmates, especially as a source of information on alternatives.

On an absolute basis, our data do not mean that inmates cope well with their problems inside of prison, but rather that they are relatively more effective than on the outside. With the serious and difficult problems they face, this may be very fortunate, considering the likely effects if inmates coped as poorly in prison as on the outside; if they did, the statistics for violence, disorder, suicide, depression, illness, and other evidence of maladjustment might be even worse than at present.

It should also be clear that to cope relatively well is not to cope absolutely well. Our ratings of efficacy were based on the likely usefulness of responses relative to the circumstances and the available alternatives. It was still the case that some subjects coped much better than others, and some unfortunately coped very poorly in prison. We saw responses of "giving up" with an unfortunate frequency, situations in which subjects said that they didn't see anything they could do about a problem, and that their only alternative was to desensitize themselves to the pain they received. Moreover, the evidence of emotional distress reviewed earlier shows how serious are the results of failures to cope with one's problems in prison.

We would argue that the conditions of imprisonment ultimately limit coping ability, because they make it difficult for inmates to acquire superior sorts of responses and strategies for dealing with problems. If most prisoners cope successfully, it is because prisons are structured in a way that makes their established coping skills relatively more appropriate. On the other hand, this very appropriateness of conditions to the established patterns of inmates will serve to decrease the pressure for change, and will reinforce old habits.

In many ways, imprisonment weakens the normal contingencies between actions and consequences. For example, our inmates were ensured that basic physical needs would be provided, almost regardless of their behavior. This dissociation between behavior and ensuing events removes much of the feedback for poor coping and the impetus for change. In effect, inmates are insulated from the demands for choices and decisions that ordinary life imposes, and one cannot easily learn to deal with situations without experiencing them.

Thus, we are led to conclude that inmates cope relatively better in prison than on the outside, and this helps most of them to weather the experience better than one might have expected. However, examination of the specifics of their coping behavior shows little real difference from what they did on the outside. Imprisonment does not seem to change overall coping skills in any significant ways.

As a result, we again see how subjects are likely to fall back into old patterns of behavior when they are released to a world of fewer constraints and greater choices. Using the entire pattern of evidence, the most supportable summary statement is that imprisonment does very little to affect the coping process directly, and we would expect that it would have no beneficial effect on the ability to cope with life on the outside.

This does not mean that imprisonment can have no effect at all on coping. Since it deprives inmates of outside experience, it might even be harmful and interfere with the developmental process that allows people to learn to cope better. Moreover, we know that the persistence of any behavior is a function of the amount of practice. If prisons allow or even encourage the repetition of behavior patterns that were maladaptive on the outside, then they may indirectly strengthen them. When we consider these arguments, we are reminded of our finding that those with the greatest experience in prison are the least effective in coping outside of prison.

Coping and Previous Imprisonment

In the previous chapter, we considered the role of the coping process in the occurrence of criminal behavior. In that discussion, we outlined some competing explanations, which should be reviewed in light of the evidence here.

One hypothesis would say that the match between coping skills and the conditions of prison is the result of previous imprisonment. By this argument, inmates learn certain ways of dealing with the world while they are in prison. When they are on the outside they behave as they did in prison, and they thus cope poorly because the behaviors they learned in prison are maladaptive in other situations. Thus, this position predicts that inmates with previous prison experience will cope better in prison than others with no prior experience, because their behavior developed as adaptations to imprisonment, although the reverse should be the case on the outside. We examined our data to test this prediction.

What appeared was that inmates without previous prison experience actually seemed to cope better than those who had such experience. For example, using the partitions of the efficacy scale explained previously, we classified 49% of the first offenders as having good coping skills, but only 24% of those with 24 months or more of previous imprisonment. Overall, the negative correlation between the amount of prior imprisonment and coping efficacy was statistically significant ($r = -.23$, $p < .01$) although it was not very large. This result is clearly opposite in direction to the prediction.

In contrast, the coping–criminality hypothesis predicts that poor coping is a major part of what distinguishes habitual offenders from others. Since we used the same scale in assessing coping efficacy both inside and outside of prison, we would expect similar negative correlations between prior criminal records and coping efficacy in both cases.

Thus, we are led to conclude that the evidence clearly favors the coping–criminality model. On the basis of all of the data in this chapter, we can argue that the behaviors involved in what we consider to be good coping are not acquired in prison.

8
The Impact of Imprisonment II—Changes over Time

The material in the preceding two chapters has shown that prison presents a strong challenge to the best of coping resources, but at the same time it also contains restrictions that facilitate at least a mediocre level of coping. From this, one might expect that most inmates would after some time become reasonably well adjusted, and show little in the way of disturbance, either emotionally or behaviorally. However, such an expectation is in contrast with other results from chapter 6 showing a large proportion of subjects suffering from strong emotional distress in prison.

All of the data presented in chapters 6 and 7 was gathered at the first interview, shortly after the beginning of subjects' terms. In this chapter we will consider the results from the two followup interviews, and look at the changes that occurred over time in prison. This will clarify a number of issues, including the apparent contradiction above.

Test-Retest Correlations

One issue that must be addressed before looking at changes is the reliability and stability of our measures across time. Following conventions for assessing this question, we calculated the correlations for each repeated measure across the three assessments. These correlations across assessments can be used to measure the reliability of measures, as well as the extent to which individuals varied (and varied in the same ways) across time.

The test-retest values for a variety of our important measures are included in Table A2 in the Appendix. The correlations vary in size, with most in the intermediate range from about .35 to .65. These values may reflect in part the unreliability of the scales used. However, it had been previously shown that the scoring is at least reasonably reliable for most of our measures. As discussed earlier, most of the questionnaires selected had been well standardized and tested; we had also checked the test-retest reliabilities of most of our interview questions in preliminary work (Zamble and Porporino, 1980) and found them to be at or above accepted levels of reliability.

Given that the correlations across interviews for our own measures were comparable to those from the widely used scales such as the Beck Depression Inventory or the State Trait Anxiety Inventory, we conclude that the correlations do not show any substantial unreliability of our measures. As would be expected with any pattern of individual changes, the correlations generally diminish over time, with the smallest values between the first and last interviews, i.e., the longest time span within the study.

Thus, we conclude that the obtained pattern of test-retest correlations indicates that the ordering of individuals across time was only moderately stable, with significant rearrangement occurring during the course of the study. This leads us to be cautious in substituting repeated measures taken at different times one for another. However, it also indicates that there is a great deal of individual variation in the process of adaptation and/or change over time in prison. This confirms the logic of the arguments for our choice of a longitudinal design, and it also shows that there is a good range of individual variability against which to test how well measures from any testing occasion will work to predict behavior on subsequent occasions.

Short-Term Changes

GENERAL LIFESTYLE AND BEHAVIOR PATTERNS

At the first interview, most subjects had been in their assigned institutions only a few weeks, and they had not yet become totally accustomed to their new environment. Although they almost all had jobs, many of them saw their positions as temporary. Although they spent time socializing, they had not had time to develop firm new relationships. Although the majority wanted to improve themselves during their term in prison, few had formulated clear plans.

In addition, their integration into ordinary institutional procedures and routines was incomplete. Payment of work stipends and access to canteen privileges had not yet been implemented for many. Visits from the outside were usually not yet possible, and mail was still catching up. All of these accompaniments of a new term were added to the usual problems and deprivations of imprisonment. The result was much distress, as indexed by such emotional states as depression and anxiety.

At the second interview, 14 to 16 weeks later, we surveyed most of the same areas. By that time inmates seemed to have settled into regular patterns of living within their various institutions. For the most part the patterns seen at the first interview remained, but some behaviors had changed, in directions that the discussion in the preceding chapters would lead one to expect. Table 8.1 shows values at the second interview and indicates changes from what we had seen earlier.

TABLE 8.1. Measures of specific behaviors related to use of time in prison (at second interview).

Variable	Value at I.2	Change from I.1
Time use categories—mean proportion of time in:		
Work	.27	− .03
Socializing	.24	+ .01
Passive activity	.23	+ .05
Sports and hobbies	.09	− .02
Visits and letters	.04	− .01
Group meetings	.02	—
Other things	.11	—
Employment		
Percent who have a job in the institution	92.3	−3.9
Mean rating of job (0–100)	70.9	—[a]
Socialization		
Mean number of friends	2.2	+0.5
Percent with no (0) friends	30.2	−9.6
Percent met majority of friends during term	43.2	−3.1
Pattern of socialization		
Stay on my own	37.7	−5.2
With a few friends	35.4	+3.8
In a larger group, or floating	22.3	+1.5
Mean percent of optional time spent in cell	30.6	+0.7
Percent specifying majority of optional time in cell	20.2	−10.1
Percent specifying no (0) optional time in cell	20.9	+0.4
Outside contacts		
Mean number of visits received (month)	1.9	+0.9
Percent with no (0) visits	46.2	+7.6
Mean number of visits desired (month)	4.7	+2.5
Percent with no (0) visits desired	27.1	+8.5
Mean number of letters received (month)	12.4	+9.0
Percent with no (0) letters	7.8	+1.5
Mean number of letters desired (month)	19.4	+13.1
Percent with no (0) letters desired	7.8	−0.6
Mean frequency of reading or listening to news (wk)	7.5	−0.3
Percent never reading or listening to news	23.8	+3.5
Time framing		
Mean frequency of thoughts of future (day/month)	17.5	—[a]
Mean frequency of thoughts of past (days/month)	12.0	—[a]

[a] Item was either not measured on the previous occasion, or its scaling was incompatible with that in measurements on this occasion, and direct comparison is not possible.

The pattern of time allocation was very similar to that from the first interview. Only the time devoted to passive activities showed a substantial difference, increasing by an amount that was statistically significant ($t = 2.74$, $p < .01$). No other category changed significantly. As subjects' status became regularized, they gained full access to the facilities that existed within each institution, such as institutional "radio" transmissions and communal television rooms. In addition, as they became familiar with (and familiar to) the rest of the inmate population, they lost most of the hesitancy they had reported about exposing themselves to communal facilities. By the end of 4 months, they were spending as much time in passive viewing or listening as in general socialization.

If the general pattern of time usage was relatively stable, there were some changes in activities within categories. While almost all were still in jobs or training programs, 43% had changed situations since the first interview, a high rate of change. Most of the switches had been requested to match work preferences, and the result was that most were quite satisfied with their employment. When we asked subjects to rate their jobs on a scale from 0 to 100, the mean rating was 71. Many remarked that their work was the most rewarding part of their lives in prison, and a substantial number would have liked more work to do.

Similarly, there were some changes in the pattern of socialization, if not in the overall time devoted to it. For example, the mean number of friends was up by about 30%, more inmates than previously said that they had close friends within their institution, and fewer said that they lived mostly on their own. Although none of these measures are critical alone, together they show that inmates had established new friendships to replace those they left behind. If the amount of socialization did not change much over time, relationships did move in the direction of greater permanence.

Thus, the pattern of subjects' lives had changed little overall from that at the original interview. However, this should not be construed as a result of any deliberate choice on their part, for most still reported a lack of any planning. As before, most said that they lived day by day. To get some additional detail, we asked if they planned their time within days: 62% said that they did not even do this, but rather they "just let things happen." Most of our subjects seemed to drift through their time, and in this they had changed little from the outside.

The one area in which there was considerable change was in the amount of contact with individuals on the outside. The number of letters and visits both showed significant increases (for letters, $t = 8.56$, $p < .001$; for visits, $t = 3.45$, $p < .001$). By the time of the second interview, subjects were corresponding with an average of 4.8 people on the outside. Interestingly, the increases in actual contacts seemed only to whet the appetite for more, and the number of visits and letters desired both more than doubled (for visits, $t = 3.89$, $p < .001$; for letters, $t = 7.86$, $p < .001$).

Still, there were some who had or desired little or no contact with people on the outside: a few received no letters at all, and almost half had no visits. Indeed, the proportions of those who either received or desired no visits at all had both risen somewhat from levels at the first interview. Thus, a significant minority of prisoners was still largely cut off from outside contacts.

For the majority, it had taken some time for mail addresses to be forwarded, for lists of visitors to be approved, etc., but this had occurred

TABLE 8.2. Common problem categories inside prison at follow-up interviews

	Percentage of subjects	
Category	Intv'w 2	Intv'w 3
1. Missing family or friends	83	77
2. Missing freedom	49	41
3. Missing specific object or activity	42	46
4. Conflicts with other inmates	26	23
5. Regrets or troubling thoughts about past	25	18
6. Concern re future, esp. life after release	44	42
7. Boredom	22	15
8. Cell conditions (privacy, noise, etc.)	15	31
9. Medical services	17	23
10. Lack of staff support or help	17	12
11. Concern about personal safety	7	9
12. Lack of desired programs or facilities	7	14

before the second interview. The lack of contact with the outside had been one of the major sources of stress at the beginning of the term, so these changes ought to have led to some improvement in emotional state. We will consider such changes shortly.

PROBLEMS AND COPING

We also looked at how the perceptions of problems and the responses to them changed by the time of the second interview. As at the first interview, each subject provided us with an ordered list of the problems he saw. The original list was not considered in the construction of the new list, so as to maximize the independence of responses.

The list of common problems at the second interview, seen in Table 8.2, was virtually unchanged from that at the first. The only problem category that changed by a nontrivial amount was concerns for the future. The proportion of the sample mentioning this problem rose from 31% to 44%, thus causing it to rise to the rank of the third most frequently cited problem. With this exception, the frequencies of listing of the other sorts of problems were virtually unchanged, showing that the problems that inmates experienced were relatively stable over the first few months of their terms.

Despite the increase in actual contacts with people on the outside, problems in missing family or friends were listed by 83% of the sample. Apparently, a limited amount of contact only increased the salience of the deprivation experienced. We had measured both actual and desired rates of contact, and it appeared that as the actual amounts increased so did the desired amounts, in almost the same proportions: the desired number of letters tripled, and the desired number of visits doubled. As a result, the absolute disparities between desires and actuality increased.

We also compared the two lists from each individual, to assess the degree of stability. At the interview the lists were compared, and we asked the subject about the reasons for any changes; if we were unsure whether items on the two lists were the same, we asked subjects to tell us whether they were different statements of the same problem, or whether they should be counted as different problems. With this information, we calculated that just under half of all the problems specified at the second interview were continuations of problems previously listed. Interestingly, the higher a problem ranked on a subject's list, the more likely was it listed for the second time. Thus, 59% of the highest ranked problems had been among the top five at the beginning of the term, but only 23% of problems ranked fifth.

Reasons for changes were usually clear. For about half of the changes the problem no longer existed, either because the situation had changed or because the subject's reaction to it was different. In only 2% of the discrepant cases did subjects say that an item omitted from the second list had been forgotten, a good indication of the thoroughness and reliability of the problem-generating procedure.

Thus, there was good consistency in the perceived problems of inmates across time, both across the entire sample and within individuals. This supports our argument that the common problems, experienced by inmates in prison are largely determined by the prevailing conditions. As conditions remained largely constant, so did the problems, especially for the aggregate of prisoners. In life generally, we would expect as much. Despite the passage of time, one's most troublesome problems tend to persist. In prison this is probably even more the case.

If subjects' problems remain very much the same, then finding ways of successfully coping with them is all the more important. The persistence of problems would also give an inmate more practice in dealing with particular situations, so we would expect improvement in coping over time.

This did not appear to have been the case. When we assessed coping at the second interview, the various measures showed little change from their previous levels. Using the same classification of responses as before, there was some switching within the cognitive control classifications, from Self-control to Re-evaluation, as can be seen in Table 8.3, but the total of the two categories remained about the same. There was also an increase again in the use of Palliatives, and much more reported use of Drug-taking, the latter presumably reflecting access gained after greater familiarity with local sources of supply.

However, no measures of coping categories at the second interview showed changes from the first interview comparable to the differences between values for life outside of prison and life within prison at the first interview. On our measures of the effectiveness of coping, there was also little change. For example, the mean level on the efficacy scale was 12.0, only trivially higher than at the first interview.

As discussed earlier, there are some reasons to expect that inmates

TABLE 8.3. Coping modes used in prison (at second interview).

Category	Percentage of subjects using	Change in Percentage from interview 1
None (giving up)	4	−4
Reactive Problem-oriented	96	0
Avoidance	51	+1
Escape	55	−6
Palliative	75	+13
Social Support	25	+4
Anticipatory Problem-oriented	9	−7
Reinterpretive (Re-evaluation)	35	+12
Reinterpretive (Self-control)	19	−13
Substitution	23	+5
Drug-taking	15	+12

might develop the ability to cope with imprisonment over time in prison. This did not happen, at least in the short term. A better judgment can be made in a few pages when we consider the data from the final interview, but we can at least say here that if inmates learn to cope with prison from direct experience they do not do so very quickly. In short, what we saw after an interval of 4 months was that inmates' problems remained pretty much the same, and so did their ways of coping with those problems.

EMOTIONAL ADJUSTMENT

At the first interview we had found evidence that strong emotional distress was widespread within the sample, with an alarming number of inmates suffering from either depression or anxiety or both. The same measures were repeated at the second interview, with the results shown in Table 8.4. As can be seen, scores improved considerably on almost all of our principal measures of emotional state. For example, the average score on the Spielberger State Anxiety Inventory had dropped significantly, to 43.3. ($t = 3.83$, $p < .001$). So did the scores on the Beck Depression Inventory ($t = 4.96$, $p < .001$) where the mean fell to 10.1, just above the range considered normal. The number of subjects with scores indicative of moderate or severe depression had fallen by more than 40%.

Other measures showed similar trends. Only the reported frequency of anger increased ($t = 2.39$, $p < .05$) and this is probably understandable when we consider that inmates' anger was usually focused and specific to conditions they faced, in contrast to depression, hopelessness, and anxiety, which were generally felt as diffuse and pervasive.

Thus, 3 months later there was generally some amelioration of the emotional disturbances seen at the beginning of the term. We should not overstate these changes, for average measures of emotional distress were still elevated, and a significant minority of subjects were still suffering. Even

TABLE 8.4. Measures of emotional state and motivations to change in prison (at second interview).

Variable	Value at I.2	Change from I.1
General appraisals		
Mean general rating of quality of life (0–100)	38.5	+3.1
Percent rating quality of life at 50 or below	79.7	−0.3
Percent specifying "No (0) positive things here"	61.2	+2.9
Emotions		
Percent with self-reported sleeping problems	40.8	−7.7
Mean frequency of emotion (week, self-report)		
Depression	2.9	−0.1
Anger	2.3	+0.4
Anxiety	2.4	−0.4
Guilt feelings	1.3	−0.2
Boredom	3.5	−0.6
Loneliness	4.0	—[a]
Percent reporting no (0):		
Depression	25.6	−4.5
Anger	34.6	−6.0
Anxiety	46.9	+11.8
Guilt feelings	69.2	+5.2
Boredom	33.8	−1.8
Loneliness	25.4	—[a]
Mean score on Beck Depression Inventory	10.1	−2.9
Mean score on Spielberger State Anxiety Inventory	43.4	−3.4
Mean score on Hopelessness Scale	2.9	−1.8
Frequency of missing people from outside—percent specifying:		
All of the time	32.8	−6.4
Most of the time	44.8	+8.0
Sometimes	12.0	−2.4
Rarely	5.6	+2.4
Never	4.8	−1.6
Planning		
Percent reporting general plan for doing time	85.8	+2.3
Percent reporting having goal for term	68.0	−12.5
Percent specifying that goal is educ'n or training	54.9	−19.9
Percent specifying that goal is behavior change	5.3	−8.3
Percent reporting choosing job for self-improvement	45.0	−15.3
Percent living day-by-day (vs planning time)	78.3	−0.7
Attempts to control thoughts—percent saying:		
Try to think about things	47.5	+10.2
Try not to think about things	27.5	+0.2
Just let thoughts happen	25.0	−10.5
Cognitions		
Mean score on Prison Control scale	100.2	—[a]
Mean score on Prison Problems scale	56.8	—[a]

[a] Not measured on the previous occasion.

more, for every three subjects who improved, one had become worse, and 5–8% of subjects had increases of over 6 points in their scores on the Beck Depression Inventory. Still, there was no question that the mood of the average subject was better at the second interview.

This indicates to us that much of the distress seen at the first interview was the result of the shock and disruption at the beginning of a prison term. At that time, inmates are still getting over the impact of their conviction and sentencing, in addition to all of the changes consequent on a new term in the penitentiary. However, with the passage of time the painful events preceding imprisonment become more distant; fortunately, memories of unpleasant experiences fade more quickly than others. Even more, the shock, disruption, and novelty of a new term in prison after a while turn into the familiarity and boredom of consistent routine. Even the worst of situations seems less devastating after one has had a chance to get used to it. For example, at the second interview the number of subjects who reported feeling totally unable to deal with any problem had fallen to half of what it was originally, even though the problems were often the same.

This does not mean that inmates become content with their lot, for certainly the increased frequency of angry episodes belies this, and their ratings of the quality of their lives were unchanged. Rather, the initial shock dissipated and left them to begin drifting through their time. If our prisons do little to help to ameliorate the initial emotional impact on prisoners, it is fortunate that the effects begin to dissipate over time.

The Closing Window

If the impact of the beginning of the term included a large amount of emotional discomfort, it had some potentially beneficial aspects as well. The disruption of old patterns had produced some commitment by subjects to change their lives. We could see it in subjects' expressed desires for self-improvement, in their choice of jobs, and in a variety of other related measures. We considered this resolution a real opportunity to effect changes in their behavior.

However, if much of the initial impact on emotional states had dissipated in the interval before the second interview, the resolution to change appears to have undergone the same decay. This may be seen in the measures under the heading of Planning in Table 8.4. For example, the original 60% who said that they had chosen their job assignment for self-improvement had dropped to 45%, as more subjects had begun to choose their positions for advantages within the institutions than previously. Similarly, fewer expressed goals for their terms, and those who did were less likely to specify goals of educational or behavioral improvement.

Other measures not shown in the table confirmed the same sort of trend. For example, when we asked subjects about their general plans for their terms, we found that the great majority reported having some such plan, but of these 34% specified that the plan was to "keep busy," 17% wanted only to "stay out of trouble," and only 18% wanted to achieve some specific objective. Their "plans" had become mostly strategies for dealing with the routine of imprisonment.

In summary, as the undesirable effects of the beginning of the term began to dissipate, so did some of the more favorable components. We might also mention that the observed increase in the frequency of anger would present another new obstacle to change, for angry men are hard to reform. Thus, it appears that the original desirable effects were a time-limited window of opportunity. We believe that at the beginning of the term a great many inmates are quite receptive to change. If this is the result of their unhappiness and emotional distress at the time, it is no less real and potentially useful. However, with the passage of time, institutional routines become the reality that inmates experience, and the present reality always takes precedence. Actual disruption becomes more distant, distress lessens, and the desire for lasting change becomes a less pressing objective to be dealt with in some remote future.

It is very unfortunate that the correctional system does not take greater advantage of this window of opportunity. At present, there is no firm policy that directs when treatment will be attempted, except in isolated cases such as the treatment of sex offenders. However, there is clearly a strong bias within the system against the use of resources to treat inmates near the beginning of their terms. Part of the staff mythology is that programs will be more effective if they "wait until the inmate settles down."

Our data show how mistaken this is. If we are correct that there is a real desire for change in many prisoners at the start of their terms, then the same data which lead us to that conclusion also indicate that motivation for change dissipates as time passes and as the shock and disruption consequent on the beginning of the term turn into routine and habit.

Active treatment or rehabilitative programs aimed at changing prisoners' behavior should be initiated as close as possible to the beginning of their terms, for new behaviors can then be more easily integrated into the developing patterns of habits and cognitions. If this recommendation were followed, we believe that there would be an increase in the success of programs, as well as an alleviation of the distress that many inmates experience at the beginning of their terms. Such a change from current practice would not by itself change the amount of resources needed for treatment, but only the timing. The results should be of benefit to both staff and inmates.

Summary: Behavior and Coping After Acclimation

Although there have been a large number of claims about the supposed deleterious effects of imprisonment, hard evidence is not easy to find. One may divide the changes which are hypothesized into three general types:

intellectual, emotional, and behavioral. The data of this study are pertinent to the latter two of these categories, and, to our knowledge, they provide the first clear information on changes over the first part of a prison sentence.

From the results, we can see why there might be some confusion about whether imprisonment leads to emotional problems among prisoners. At the beginning of their terms, many subjects showed signs of emotional disturbances. For example, an alarmingly high proportion showed indications of depressive states of clinical magnitude. Thus, the initial effect of imprisonment is emotionally devastating for many offenders.

However, the other side of our results shows that much of the initial traumatic effect of imprisonment was short-lived. After a few months there was visible improvement, and we can generalize that the proportion of inmates at risk had fallen by about half. From the explanation given, we would expect that the changes would continue to develop for some time, and the data in subsequent sections will demonstrate this.

While the pattern of initial shock and gradual adjustment seems almost intuitively obvious in hindsight, it had not previously been documented very clearly; if our conclusion about emotional acclimation to imprisonment has been stated before (e.g., Sapsford, 1978, 1983) it required a great inductive leap over a field of fragmentary data. The data of this study should help to fill in some of the gaps.

It is true that there were still many subjects at the second interview who showed the need for help with emotional problems. However, this does not constitute evidence for deleterious effects of imprisonment, because there are reasons to believe that many subjects entered prison with substantial emotional problems. For example, the data on the amount of alcoholism on the outside certainly indicate the likely presence of previous depressive problems for many subjects, and a substantial number also reported previous treatment for emotional problems. Even without this evidence, our coping–criminality hypothesis almost demands that many offenders would have shown emotional disorders prior to imprisonment.

Therefore, we conclude that the amount of emotional disturbance visible at the second interview was the sum of disturbances that inmates brought with them and the remnant of the effects of the initial shock of imprisonment. The latter should disappear after the passage of more time, but because of the former we would always expect to find more emotional maladjustment in prison than in a standardized normal population.

In the ideal case, it would be definitive to have measurements of offenders' emotional states before arrest, to track the changes after arrest, trial, sentencing, and imprisonment, but this is of course practically impossible. In the absence of such data, we would argue that any conclusions about the effects of imprisonment on emotional states should be based on changes that are seen to develop over the course of time in prison. Some previous writers have observed emotional distress in prison, and in the classic fallacy of *post hoc ergo propter hoc* they have argued that what they saw was the result of imprisonment. However, with the advantage of repeated measures in a longitudinal design, we see much more evidence for improvement over time, rather than the accumulation of deleterious effects.

One may wonder why this occurred. We believe that an examination of the reasons can be quite revealing about the way inmates experience imprisonment.

As we have stated repeatedly, at the beginning of a term in prison a person is presented with a great variety of new conditions. He may experience some things as oppressive, and the novelty emphasizes their effect. However, he is also subject to the dulling routine of prison as soon as he arrives. Aside from the diversions that prisoners invent for themselves, each day is like any other. After a while, the routines become familiar, and then monotonous. Although the monotony and boredom may seem to many inmates to be problems in their own right, they serve to lower arousal levels and lull people into lassitude and stolid adherence to the daily routine. If offenders had concentrated their attention on the present while on the outside, after a while in prison they become even more locked into a permanent focus on the present moment.

So the routine of imprisonment dulls inmates' perceptions and lulls them into its own rhythm. At the same time, their problems remain and do not change much over time. Human beings show a remarkable capacity to adjust to all sorts of conditions. Research on such phenomena as adaptation levels (Helson, 1964) shows that people adjust to changes in environmental events in such a way that after some time the new levels are used as norms for comparisons. We would argue that prisoners adjust in the same way, so that after a while the conditions they see in prison come to seem normal. With novelty and surprise gone, deprivations and restrictions no longer evoke their original responses, and emotional reactions begin to fall to normal levels.

Nothing ever changes here. You do the same things every day, see the same faces, eat the same meals. Sometimes I imagine that my mind could go to sleep for a year or two, while my body stayed here. When I'd awake nothing would be different, maybe nobody would even notice. I get less upset than I used to.

The commonest concern that inmates told us regarding their immediate future was about avoiding "institutionalization." On the basis of the argument above, we can understand this concern. The return to more normal levels of emotional reactivity after a few months in prison is not accomplished by solution of problems, nor by personal growth, but by a numbness brought on by routine and constancy. It is probably this lowering of reactivity which some inmates sense, and which they fear will grow until it dulls other faculties as well.

(Fortunately, evidence from other studies shows fairly well that general deterioration does not occur, despite the fears popularized by writers such as Cohen and Taylor (1981). For example, Banister, Smith, Heskin, and Bolton (1973) show that intellectual abilities are not impaired by imprisonment. A survey of the literature that comes to a similar conclusion may be seen in Walker (1983).)

One other line of argument follows from the data of the second interview. While we have commented at length on the differences between measures at the first interview and those 4 months later, we have not discussed the implications of the similarities. Indeed, no changes were visible in the great majority of measures. This could mean that our measures are insensitive to change. However, in view of the sizeable differences using the same measures between the results for inside prison and those for life on the outside, we find such an explanation very unlikely.

Rather, we think that the lack of change on most behavioral measures is quite significant, for it shows how quickly the routine of life in prison is established. It also leads us to argue that there is very little learning involved in the behavioral adaptation to imprisonment. Learning normally shows itself over a period of time, during which a set of constraints or contingencies lead to progressive changes in behavior. In contrast, in the case of imprisonment the changes seem to be sudden and complete within a short period. Therefore, we would argue that the differences from the outside are forced and inevitable responses to the special conditions of imprisonment, and that any learning that occurs is minimal.

The upshot of this argument is the prediction that the changes in behavior that occur in prison are likely to be immediately reversed after inmates are released. If the adaptation is forced by the environment and not by learning, then the effects will last only as long as the originating conditions. Thus, we can explain why it is that imprisonment does not lead to much in the way of permanent changes in the behavior of offenders. We shall return to this topic also at a later point.

One Year Later

NEW CHANGES

The final interview and testing were done approximately one year after the second, and thus almost a year and a half after the beginning of subjects' sentences. Although the sample was essentially the same for the first two interviews, by the time of the third interview some attrition had occurred, as subjects in the short- and medium-term groups were released, and only about 100 subjects were available for the final interview.

We had chosen the intervals for the study so as to allow the final interview just before the time of mandatory release (two-thirds of the sentence) but subjects became unavailable for a variety of reasons, mostly parole or early release programs. Therefore, overall means from the final interview must be interpreted cautiously. Any conclusions that we make concerning changes over the term are based on comparisons of scores only for the subjects who completed the third interview. This avoids the distortions that might come from comparing the results of different sets of subjects, but it does limit the generality. Still, any conclusions we make about changes that occur over time in prison should be valid.

Despite the problem of attrition, the pattern of results we saw at the third interview was very similar to what we had seen earlier in the term. Not many things had changed. Where there were differences from the second interview, they were mostly the continuation of changes seen from the first interview to the second. Values on all interviews for the variety of measures presented earlier for the first two interviews can be seen in Tables 8.5 and 8.6. (It should be noted that the numbers in these tables are based only on the subjects who completed the final interview, so in some cases they vary slightly from figures cited previously for the larger samples in the first two interviews.)

Only among the variables measuring socialization did there appear to be some new changes. For the most part, the breakdown of time into our various categories was the same as at the second interview. However, there was a significant decrease in the time spent socializing from that seen before, to a mean level of 3.3 hours daily from the 4.2 at the second interview $(t = 2.13, p < .05)$. The decrease is also significant when compared to the first interview $(t = 2.15, p < .05)$.

This change was mirrored in almost all of our other indicators of social interactions. For example, the mean number of friends showed a substantial and significant decrease from the second interview $(t = 2.92, p < .01)$. The mean time that subjects spent in their own cells, that is, when they chose some solitary activity in preference to socializing, rose by about one-quarter $(t = 2.45, p < .05)$. The proportion of subjects who specified that they chose to spend their time mostly on their own increased to a clear majority.

Thus, those inmates who remained after about a year and a half had begun to spend more time on their own. From the data and from their responses, it does not appear that they were avoiding social activities per se, but they did now prefer other ways of spending their time.

At the same time, changes in the amount of socialization with other inmates were not accompanied by decreases in contact with the outside, for measures of outside contact showed no changes from levels at the second interview. In other areas as well, there were no apparent differences from what we had seen a year previously.

CONTINUING CHANGES

At the second interview, changes in two major areas were apparent: an improvement in the emotional distress seen at the beginning of the term,

TABLE 8.5. Measures of specific behaviors related to use of time in prison (across all interviews)[a]

Variable	I1	I2	I3
Time use categories—mean proportion of time in:			
Work	.30	.26	.30
Socializing	.24	.24	.20
Passive activity	.19	.25	.24
Sports and hobbies	.10	.09	.11
Visits and letters	.05	.04	.04
Group meetings	.02	.02	.02
Other things	.10	.10	.09
Employment			
Percent who have a job in the institution	96.1	93.8	94.8
Mean rating of job (0–100)	—[b]	69.0	75.9
Socialization			
Mean number of friends	1.9	2.1	1.5
Percent with no (0) friends	38.1	30.2	39.2
Percent met majority of friends during term	43.3	43.9	62.7
Pattern of socialization			
Percent stay on my own	38.1	41.2	56.7
Percent with a few friends	36.1	38.1	28.9
Percent in a larger group, or floating	23.7	15.5	14.4
Mean percent of optional time spent in cell	30.1	29.4	38.3
Percent specifying majority of optional time in cell	19.8	19.8	28.6
Percent specifying no (0) optional time in cell	29.2	21.9	18.7
Outside contacts			
Mean number of visits received (month)	0.9	1.5	1.3
Percent with no (0) visits	39.6	49.5	48.5
Mean number of visits desired (month)	2.4	4.7	2.9
Percent with no (0) visits desired	13.7	26.0	34.0
Mean number of letters received (month)	3.4	11.8	12.5
Percent with no (0) letters	14.4	6.3	15.5
Mean number of letters desired (month)	6.0	19.8	19.9
Percent with no (0) letters desired	8.4	7.3	10.4
Mean frequency of reading or listening to news (wk)	7.7	7.7	8.5
Percent never reading or listening to news	20.6	20.6	9.3
Time framing			
Mean frequency of thoughts of future (days/month)	—[b]	16.6	—[b]
Mean frequency of thoughts of future in prison	—[b]	—[b]	5.8
Mean frequency of thoughts of future outside	—[b]	—[b]	15.7
Mean frequency of thoughts of past	—[b]	12.0	10.4

[a] Values for first and second testings may differ from those in earlier tables, since only subjects who were tested all 3 times are included here, in order to provide more accurate comparisons.
[b] Item was either not measured on the given occasion, or its scaling was incompatible with other measurements and direct comparison is not possible.

TABLE 8.6. Measures of emotional state and motivations to change in prison (across all interviews).[a]

	Value at		
Variable	I1	I2	I3
General appraisals			
Mean general rating of quality of life (0–100)	35.2	38.7	37.2
Percent rating quality of life 50 or below	82.1	82.1	81.3
Percent specifying "No (0) positive things here"	38.5	35.4	35.1
Emotions			
Percent with self-reported sleeping problems	48.5	43.3	29.2
Mean frequency of emotion (week, self-report)			
Depression	3.2	2.9	2.2
Anger	1.9	2.4	2.4
Anxiety	2.8	2.4	1.9
Guilt feelings	1.4	1.2	0.5
Boredom	4.0	3.5	3.5
Loneliness	—[b]	4.2	4.1
Percent reporting no (0)			
Depression	28.9	24.7	34.0
Anger	39.2	29.9	32.3
Anxiety	35.4	48.5	56.7
Guilt feelings	69.1	67.0	79.4
Boredom	33.0	30.9	27.8
Loneliness	—[b]	21.6	15.5
Mean score on Beck Depression Inventory	13.2	10.4	10.4
Mean score on Spielberger State Anxiety Invnt'y	46.2	43.4	41.6
Mean score on Hopelessness Scale	5.2	3.1	3.6
Mean score on Self-Esteem Scale	5.9	—[b]	7.5
Frequency of missing people from outside—percent specifying:			
All of the time	34.4	29.3	25.8
Most of the time	38.9	44.6	44.3
Sometimes	16.7	13.0	10.3
Rarely	4.4	7.6	12.4
Never	5.5	5.4	7.2
Planning			
Percent reporting general plan for doing time	82.5	85.1	87.6
Percent reporting having goal for term	79.3	71.6	61.9
Percent specifying having goal educ'n or training	58.6	62.1	40.6
Percent specifying having goal bhv'r change	10.9	4.2	5.2
Percent choosing job for self-improvement	60.6	—[b]	33.0
Percent planning time (vs living day-by-day)	22.0	21.9	21.3
Attempts to control thoughts—percent saying:			
Try to think about things	35.9	46.1	54.9
Try not to think about things	28.2	30.3	24.2
Just let thoughts happen	35.9	23.6	20.9
Cognitions			
Mean score on Prison Control Scale	—[b]	98.7	99.9
Mean score on Prison Problems Scale	—[b]	58.4	59.3
Mean score on Internal-External Scale (external)	48.2	—[b]	51.5
Mean Attitudes Toward Criminal Justice System	72.2	—[b]	76.5

TABLE 8.6. (*continued*)

	Value at		
Variable	I1	I2	I3
Self-categorizations			
Doing time (avoid trouble, get out soon)	37.5	—[b]	56.3
Gleaning (better myself, profit from the time)	52.1	—[b]	31.3
Jailing (forget the outside, have a good time)	10.4	—[b]	12.5

[a] Values for first and second testings may differ from those in earlier tables, since only subjects who were tested all 3 times are included here, in order to provide more accurate comparisons.
[b] Item was either not measured on the given occasion, or its scaling was incompatible with other measurements and direct comparison is not possible.

and a concomitant decay of the motivation to change that had also been visible.

Both of these sorts of changes continued in the year before the third interview. As can be seen in Table 8.6, the reported frequencies of episodes of depression, anxiety, and guilt all continued to decrease. The differences from the levels at the second interview were significant for the State Anxiety Scale ($t = 2.14$, $p < .05$) and for the frequency of guilt feelings ($t = 2.29$, $p < .05$), which dropped to a nearly invisible level, although the further changes in the other measures of current emotional states did not reach statistical reliability. There were also significant improvements from the first interview on Self-Esteem ($t = 5.06$, $p < .001$), which was not included in the second test battery. Thus, there were continuing reductions in most measures of dysphoric emotional states.

The exceptions are revealing. The frequency of anger remained unchanged, not surprising to us because we believe that anger is evoked by many everyday events within prison. And, of course, loneliness and boredom were also as high as before, because they are evoked by the unalterable absence of certain things or people.

Thus, by the third interview, most subjects had recovered from the emotional trauma seen at the start of their terms. However, we should also note that the mean levels on some emotional indices were probably still elevated, even though they had dropped to within the normal (subclinical) range.

There are reasons to expect that a further follow-up study would show a continuing trend for decreases in dysphoria. For example, Sapsford (1978) found differences in Hopelessness—a scale we also used—between groups of inmates who had served 15 months and 6 years, in a cross-sectional design. Considering that his first group had served about the same amount of time as inmates at our final interview, his data suggest that the process of emotional adjustment continues over several years.

Another reason for the same expectation is based on our observations of how slowly the wheels of justice grind. Even at our third interview, a year and a half after committal to the penitentiary, only about half of subjects' appeals had been adjudicated. It is easy to understand how a prisoner with an appeal pending could exist in a psychological limbo, and why he might not have reached any emotional equilibrium.

In any case, we are strengthened in the conclusion that the initial emotional disturbance produced by imprisonment is generally impermanent. At the same time, there is also further evidence that the window of opportunity for real behavior reform was lost. For example, the proportion of subjects at the last interview who reported having chosen their prison employment because of the opportunity for self-improvement fell to half of that at the first interview. Using Irwin's categories, the proportion of inmates who identified themselves as "gleaners" fell from 52% at the first interview to 31% at the third. Other indices showed similar trends. The evidence of motivation for self-improvement and personal change had almost disappeared.

In short, with the shock of the beginning of the term behind them, the majority of inmates seemed to be drifting through time. Only 15% had a specific plan to achieve some objective while in prison. More than three-quarters said that they "just let things happen" rather than even planning their time within a day. Clearly, after a while most were living moment by moment.

This was not only the case for their management of their present time, but the same could be seen in planning for the future. Since release was then far in the future for most subjects who remained in prison, thinking of the future was mostly a means of escape akin to daydreaming or fantasizing. When we asked for future plans, most seemed to consist of fanciful objectives without any concrete plans, e.g., "I will get married, get a good job, settle down, and never come back here—but I'll figure out the details once I get out there." Given the time before release, perhaps there was no real point in making detailed plans for the future, but we can see how the drift through time included both present and future.

One final piece of information should be included in this section. Although subjects' emotional reactions to imprisonment had improved over time, their evaluations of prison conditions were no higher. For example, their mean rating of the quality of prison life remained low and unchanged across interviews. Clearly, prisoners did not feel that things had improved in their lives, nor had they lost their critical capacities. Instead, the potential stress they experienced had been mitigated by repetition, regularity, and the constancy of the prison environment. In this, their exclusive focus on their concrete present reality may have been central.

PROBLEMS AND COPING

If general behavior patterns and lifestyle changed little in the year before our last interview, the problems experienced by subjects were also mostly static. When we looked at the common problems cited on subjects' lists, included previously in Table 8.2, no new concerns appeared, and the proportions with problems in each of the respective categories were not much different than before.

If we consider the changes that did occur, they mostly fit the generalization that subjects were becoming more concerned with their "here and now." Thus, the frequencies of problems with cell conditions, medical services, and availability of programs and facilities, all rose, while concerns about missing family, missing freedom, and events in the past, all decreased in frequency. It would appear that the longer men live in prison, the more they restrict their concerns to the concrete present reality that it presents for them.

We also compared each subject's list to his list from the second interview, and again there was a good deal of consistency, with about the same overlap from the second to the third interview as reported earlier for that from the first to the second. Thus, there is stability in the things that inmates appraise as potentially stressful. Situations that are seen as problems at one time are likely to remain as problems, even a year later.

However, one interesting change did appear. Aside from the choices of problems, the total number of problems mentioned was higher than at the first interview ($t = 2.94, p < .01$). Thus, again we can see that the reduction in emotional distress over time in prison was not because of any improvement in inmates' appreciation of their situations.

If the types of problems seen did not change much over time, it was also the case that our measures of specific coping responses showed little change at the third interview. Overall ways of approaching problems were the same, as can be seen in Table 8.7, and we could see no real differences in the modes of coping responses that were used, except perhaps for a further increase in the use of palliatives. The mean efficacy score was 12.2,

TABLE 8.7. Coping modes used in prison (at all 3 interviews).

	Percentage of subjects using		
Category	I1	I2	I3
None (giving up)	7	2	4
Reactive Problem-oriented	99	99	98
Avoidance	53	50	47
Escape	60	54	55
Palliative	62	74	84
Social Support	25	29	27
Anticipatory Problem-oriented	14	8	10
Reinterpretive (Re-evaluation)	22	35	35
Reinterpretive (Self-control)	30	19	31
Substitution	20	25	19
Drug-taking	3	13	8
Mean total response modes	3.9	4.0	4.2

very slightly higher than at the second interview. While the changes across interviews were small, they were consistent, and as a result coping efficacy at the last interview was significantly higher than at the first ($t = 2.34$, $p < .05$); however, the increase in the mean score of 0.4 should be considered in light of a range of over 10 from the best to the worst scores, so it is really rather trivial.

The data on changes over interviews were used for one more set of analyses. As discussed earlier, some theoretical positions predict that inmates learn their maladaptive habits in prison. While we saw no evidence for such learning in our sample as a whole, the majority of subjects had had previous prison experience, so one might concentrate the search for changes on those men who had not been in prison before their current terms. In this case, the predictions would be that the changes in new inmates would be much more substantial than in those with prior prison experience. We looked for such effects within almost all of the measures that were mentioned earlier in this chapter as showing changes across the three interviews, and in some others that did not show any overall changes. There was no suggestion that there were any significant differences in the amounts of change over time that were associated with differences in prior prison experience. We must again conclude that prisons do not teach inmates to behave any more maladaptively than they do when they enter.

Summary: The Effects of Longer-Term Imprisonment

The results of the final interview provide little that is different from what we saw on earlier occasions. The two principal sorts of changes that we saw at the second interview were continued. The rhythms of subjects' lives became even more locked into institutional routines. Their chronic problems remained chronic, and while they could cope day by day, it was by yielding to (and thus reinforcing) the routines, and in narrowing their attention to the present moment. To help manage the present, they avoided the future except as a source of fantasies, and kept the past only for the comfort of some of its happier moments.

Otherwise, most aspects of their behavior had changed not at all from the beginning of their terms. The one exception to this was a substantial falloff in the amount of voluntary social interactions with other inmates. We are not sure why this happened, but the most likely explanation is that it follows from the most frequently cited problem in prison, that is, the restrictions in contact with loved ones.

When friends and lovers from the outside are missing, the only relationships available as a substitute are those with other inmates. Yet, these also are often painful because inmates have no control over transfers, releases, or other movements that can produce abrupt separations. Those with long terms told us that they avoided relationships with short-term inmates, who were bound to be released or transferred quickly, leaving them all the more open to loneliness.

It doesn't pay to get involved with people here. I was really friendly with a kid here. He was from my home town and I'd met him on the street, and he was all broken up being here. So I talked with him a lot, and taught him the ropes, nothing sexual, I felt like a big brother. Then he got transferred down to (another institution) and I felt like hell. I mean, now when I see all these other guys here they remind me I got no one I can really talk to.

At the same time, close relationships with other long-termers, suffering from the same deprivations, often intensified their own feelings of loneliness. Thus, many long-term inmates began to adopt more solitary lifestyles after a while. Their social contacts became limited and often superficial, to avoid the entanglements, obligations, and conflicts that often result from socialization in the prison, as well as to prevent further injury from loss of people to whom they were close.

Some of this may have been an unconscious adaptation to conditions, but we have reason to believe that much of it was deliberate. At each interview we asked subjects about their attempts to control their thoughts, and we saw clear changes over time that are visible in Table 8.6. Although prisoners' patterns of external behavior generally changed little over time, there was a progressive trend toward increased efforts to control thoughts. Statistically, the changes over time were significant; for example, comparing the proportions of those who said that they "tried to think about things" at the first interview and at the last, $t = 3.32$, $p < .001$. Thus, the majority of long-term prisoners had become more self-controlled in their thoughts, parallel to the way they had also become socially more self-contained. Some had become hardened, sealing off their capacities to reach outside of the present moment of the self.

If this description goes beyond the limits of our quantified data, it was clear enough at a clinical level: the pattern was often visible in the faces and demeanor of the men we interviewed, and the changes from the first to the last interviews were sometimes quite marked.

Since they emerged only at the last interview, the time span of this study was insufficient to chart much of the progress of these changes, and an interview at a later time would have been desirable. However, by the last interview we had seen the emergence of some effects that are probably characteristic of long-term imprisonment. The changes in socialization are signs of the coldness and self-containment of men who have long been cut off from intimate contacts with other people. Psychological survival was the goal, and they did manage to cope , but the cost was considerable.

9
Circumstances: Some Major Personal and Environmental Variables

In the last few chapters we have seen how the basic conditions of imprisonment act as very powerful constraints, and how they largely determine the basic pattern of inmates' behavior in prison. However, even in prison we saw much variation in behavior.

This raises some important theoretical questions. From our interactionist position, we would of course say that the obtained results show well how personal characteristics and the local environment work together to produce individual patterns of behavior. However, it might also be claimed that we have ignored the effects of many external factors that differed across subjects.

For example, we have until now ignored the effects of institutions: conditions varied enough across the institutions from which we recruited our subjects that we might have expected some systematic and sizeable effects on behavior. Similarly, we have not considered effects of major differences in inmates' personal circumstances in prison, e.g., the length of their sentences. One might expect that a person facing a long term would act differently than another who could look forward to release in a relatively short time. Thus, what we have described in the preceding sections are nonspecific effects averaged across differences in the specifics that any inmate had to face. Therefore, it is now appropriate for us to examine the influence of variables such as institutions and sentence length on the behaviors we have already described. Such an assessment comprises the subject of this chapter.

Differences Across Institutions

With our emphasis on the interactions between individuals and the events they encounter, we have assumed that the details of the actual environments are (within normal limits) relatively weak determinants of behavior and/or adaptation. Different individuals will interpret a given set of conditions in different ways, and their reactions depend on their appraisals rather than the objectively measured reality. Moreover, as we have stressed repeatedly, even knowing a person's appraisal of a situation does not allow prediction of the response, because individuals differ in the sets of responses in their repertoires.

So we predicted that, within the context of imprisonment, differences among institutions will be relatively unimportant in determining differences in inmates' behavior. The presence of a large number of sizeable institutional differences would show that this is incorrect, and invalidate at least this aspect of the theory. On the other hand, if the differences are minimal we will have additional support for our position that individual processes of appraisal and coping are more important than details of the environment.

We had previously done some analyses that evaluated these questions, looking at differences in behavior and adaptation among men in the various medium-security institutions in the Ontario region, the same as used in this study (Porporino, 1983). In the results we could see no significant differences. However, for the present analyses we reasoned that the previous comparisons may have been inadequate to reveal the important differences across institutions for statistical reasons. Using each institution as a separate level in the analyses is based on the assumption that differences among similar institutions are more important than their commonalities. Moreover, it also has the effect of greatly reducing the power of statistical tests to discriminate among alternatives.

Accordingly, we carried out a set of comparisons across the different types of institutions to which inmates in this study had been assigned. We tried to aid the power of statistical tests by reducing the number of categories in the analyses. We reasoned that the differences across institutions that would most likely affect behavior were those associated with the severity of restrictions and the degree of confinement, i.e., security levels. Thus, we combined the various institutions into four groups according to the level of custody: maximum (Millhaven); medium (Collins Bay, Joyceville, Warkworth); minimum (Bath, Pittsburgh, Frontenac, Beaver Creek); and protective custody (Kingston). Given the nonordinal nature of the categories, we used chi-square tests for the analyses.

Since our principal objective was to evaluate the effects of institutions on behavior, we planned a set of comparisons on a wide variety of measures across institutions. However, we did not expect that inmates would have been randomly assigned to institutions of different security levels. As a result, any differences we might find could be the effects of institutions, or they might instead simply reflect differences originating in the original assignment process. Thus, in order to deal with the possible confounding effects of any differences at assignment, we needed to see how the original assignmental were arranged.

Therefore, our first analyses compared background and personal history measures against the security level of the institution of original assignment, to find out on what basis the assignments had been made. Both the length of sentence and the category of the current offense differed significantly ($p < .001$) across institutional categories in the directions that one would expect. That is, longer sentences were strongly related to higher security levels, as were offenses involving violence, especially murder, which invariably resulted in assignment to maximum security. These two variables are obviously confounded statistically, and also very much redundant, since the most serious offenses are those that draw long sentences. Therefore, we considered sentence length alone as a predictor of institutional assignment, and found that we were able to correctly predict the security levels of 88% of our subjects.

At the same time, it appeared that no other background factors had been taken into account very much in assigning inmates to institutions. Certainly the previous criminal history or records of previous imprisonment had not been given much weight. If anything, there was a tendency for those in maximum security to have shorter previous criminal histories. For example, 14% of those in maximum security had 20 or more convictions on their record, compared to 39% of those in medium-security institutions.

On this evidence, we can say that assignments had been based almost entirely on consideration of the current offense and sentence. Obviously, such practices assume that these variables have a strong relationship to behavior in prison. We will examine the importance of sentence length as a determinant of prison behavior later in this chapter, and in the following chapter we will consider predictors of various measures of adaptation in prison. In anticipation of that evidence, we can say that neither sentence length nor the category of the current offense is much related to most subsequent behaviors in prison. Thus, the assignment of inmates to institutions was based on factors that are basically unrelated to subsequent behavior or adaptation in prison. This of course presents a problem for institutional procedures, but it was fortunate for us, because it means that initial assignments were not confounded with factors that affect any of our measures very much. In effect, we could proceed as though the assignments had been according to a random process.

With this information, we performed a second set of analyses, in which we looked at the effects of institutions on later behavior. For these we compared all of our measures of coping and adaptation at the final interview across the institutions in which inmates were living at that time. No significant differences were visible on any of these comparisons. Specifically, we could find no evidence that the level of security was associated with anxiety, depression, medical problems, disciplinary incidents, usage of time, mention of specific problems, the efficacy of coping, or almost anything else that we measured.

From this, one might be tempted to conclude that either our measures or the statistical comparisons we used were insensitive. However, this must be tempered by significant differences on a number of appraisal measures.

Although the behavior of inmates did not seem to be affected by institutional differences, inmates clearly perceived real differences in the harshness of conditions across levels of security. Thus, the higher the level of security, the lower inmates rated their overall quality of life ($p < .05$). Similarly, inmates in higher levels of custody were less likely to find positive things in their environments ($p < .05$), they mentioned a greater number of problems ($p < .05$), and they had higher scores on the Hopelessness Scale ($p < .05$).

Thus, inmates did perceive differences in the quality of life in different institutions. At the same time, such perceptions were not accompanied by differences in behavior or adaptation. Considering the large differences across institutions in the degree of restriction and confinement, the absence of adaptational or behavioral differences is impressive.

This outcome is consistent with our theoretical expectations. Features of the environment will affect primary appraisals, as measured by such things as the perception of an undesirable situation. However, this does not necessarily affect either secondary appraisals or the coping process. In the end, adaptation is determined by the success of coping, not the problems that are dealt with. Thus, the problems of prisoners in a maximum-security institution may be objectively more severe, but human beings are sufficiently elastic that the harsher conditions do not necessarily produce more deleterious outcomes.

Of course, this does not mean that the conditions within a prison are irrelevant, and we certainly would not want to appear to be justifying the use of severe confinement. High security levels are not only harsh and repressive, but they are also expensive and difficult to maintain. Moreover, the higher the level of security, the more different are conditions from those in the outside world. We will argue later that a major reason for the failure of prisons to change offender behavior is that they differ as much as they do from the outside world. Thus, we would conclude that high security levels are counterproductive and undesirable. However, at the same time, we can find no evidence that differences in security levels will lead to differences in how well inmates ultimately adapt.

Length of Sentence

If the details of the external environment are relatively unimportant, one might still expect that major differences in individual circumstances would show their effects. Most important among these should be the length of sentence.

Inmates in our long-term group (sentences of 10 years and up) differed from the others in that they could not realistically look forward to leaving prison within the time scale of this study, at least not by any ordinary and legal means. For most of them the earliest form of partial release (day parole) was at least several years after the final interview. In contrast, subjects in the other groups were all eligible for day parole by about the time of the third interview, and many were actually released before then. This difference in the possibility of release seemed a critical one, and one might have expected that it would affect many aspects of behavior, e.g., planning of time and concern for the future. It was also clear that long-term inmates, especially those with life sentences, are treated quite differently from others by the penitentiary system.

Therefore, we tested whether there were statistically reliable differences between subjects in the long-term group and the others, on virtually all of the measures we had taken on our several occasions. The number of differences which appeared was surprisingly small. However, some of those which did appear are quite interesting, and they appear to fall into a coherent pattern.

One set of differences shows how long-term inmates were treated differently by the prison system. For example, the great majority of them were originally assigned to maximum-security, as opposed to only a small majority of inmates with shorter sentences ($p < .001$). We have already cited this difference in the previous section, but it shows again that an inmate's current offense was the most powerful determinant of the treatment he received in the system. Not only were long-term inmates originally assigned to higher security levels, but they were also less likely to be transferred ($p < .01$) to lower security levels, and as a result they were still at higher levels a year and a half into their terms ($p < .001$).

Thus, long-term inmates were seen as greater risks by those responsible for institutional assignments and transfers. As a result, they were faced with much greater limitations of choice and opportunity than other inmates, and they had little chance of quick improvement in their circumstances. This was clearly the result of a deliberate and overt policy in the system.

We heard many times from both subjects and staff that long-term inmates were expected to "prove" themselves by maintaining good records for several years in maximum security before they would be recommended for transfers. This was much more severe than the policy for other inmates, who could expect to have a transfer to a lower security level approved after only 6 months of good conduct. Among our long-term subjects, access to vocational training or therapeutic programs was sometimes denied or postponed indefinitely on the grounds that "there will be lots of time for that later." Thus, the current situation amounts to something like double jeopardy: a person is punished for serious offenses by imposition of a long sentence, and then again by especially severe conditions of imprisonment.

When we looked for some empirical support for this policy, it did not appear. Our data showed no reliable relationships between sentence length and any measure of adaptation at the final interview, from depression to the number of disciplinary offenses during the term.

At the same time, the lack of differences in adaptation is consistent with the interpretation of the prison experience in the preceding chapters. The differences between prison and life on the outside are sufficiently large that in many respects there is a disjunction between an individual's conduct on the outside and his behavior within an institution. As a consequence, one cannot predict very well how a person will behave in prison from knowledge of a few actions on the outside. In particular, within a penitentiary population, all of whom have committed serious crimes, behavior during a term in prison cannot be predicted from measures of the seriousness of offenses, such as sentence length.

In any case, we can conclude that long-term inmates face harsher conditions than others, especially when we consider the results in the previous section showing how the perceived quality of life varies with the level of security. It is therefore to be expected that long-term inmates would show higher levels of stress, and some evidence for this did appear, especially at the first interview. For example, long-term subjects had higher scores on Hopelessness ($p < .01$) and lower scores on the Self-Esteem Scale ($p < .05$). They were also less sanguine about the future, expecting to be more depressed ($p < .01$) and to have lower feelings of well-being ($p < .05$) a year into the future.

Therefore, we can say that long-term inmates were originally showing greater stress than other inmates, although the evidence is rather weak. However, there was no evidence at all that this was followed by differences on any of the principal indicators of emotional, medical, or behavioral problems. This does not mean that inmates with long sentences were without problems at the beginning of the term, for they suffered the same disruption and ill effects as other inmates. Still, they did not appear any worse than others in the system.

One possible explanation for the absence of stronger effects at the first interview is that it might take some time for the effects of sentence length to develop. As we have already discussed, many long-term inmates had not yet begun to adjust to the reality of their sentences. The majority were actively considering or pursuing appeals, a higher proportion than inmates with shorter sentences ($p < .001$) and those who were appealing had higher expectations of the likely success of their appeals ($p < .001$). As a result, many were in a psychological and emotional limbo at the time of the first interview. If this was so, then one might expect the deleterious effects of long sentences to be delayed.

However, our follow-up interviews did not show any such effects. Rather, even the weak evidence for greater emotional problems among long-term inmates disappeared, and the few differences between groups were weak, inconsistent, and generally trivial. For example, long-term subjects reported more guilt feelings at the second interview ($p < .05$) but this might be interpreted as reasonable considering the greater gravity of their offenses. Similarly, the mean frequency of loneliness reported at the last interview was higher in the long-term group ($p < .05$), but this was likely a selection artifact.

Other than these differences, there were few significant effects of sentence length on emotional or behavioral measures after the first interview. Measures of outcomes or adaptation over the term were similarly unaffected. The only exceptions were that long-term inmates reported receiving more letters and spent more time in passive activities at the final interview ($p < .05$ for each).

Given the evidence for greater strains imposed by the system on long-term subjects, one might wonder why they did not show more ill effects. One possible reason is that they coped better. Potentially stressful situations become problems only with inadequate means of coping, and a more difficult situation need not be damaging if coping resources are adequate.

When we compared shorter-term and long-term subjects we found that the long-term group indeed had higher scores on our measure of Coping Efficacy in prison ($p < .05$). This is very unlikely to have developed in prison, and there is evidence that long-term subjects were also better at coping outside of prison. For example, they reported more use of higher-level coping strategies previous to imprisonment ($p < .01$). We can also recall that a greater proportion of the long-term subjects were imprisoned for the first time, and that coping was negatively correlated with the amount of previous imprisonment. If long-term inmates adjusted as well as others, it was because they brought better coping resources to the situation.

In summary, we found only minimal effects of sentence length on the day-to-day behavior of inmates. In this we see one more indication of how the basic conditions of imprisonment dominate other factors. One would expect a person to suffer some shock at the imposition of a long sentence, and indeed the discrepancy between the actual sentence and that expected before trial was much greater for long-term subjects than for others ($p < .001$). In addition, it seems reasonable to assume that the impact of a prison sentence on emotions and thoughts would be a simple function of the length of the sentence.

Nevertheless, we could see very little real difference attributable to sentence length. Any likely effects were lost in the general emotional and behavioral disruption at the beginning of the term. By the time those initial effects had dissipated, subjects were firmly and immovably settled into institutional routines that were not easily disrupted. Habits are usually very resistant to change once established, especially within a constant environment, so that effects which do not appear at once in prison are unlikely to appear at all. Thus, there were no appreciable differences in behavior to differentiate individuals with long terms from others.

This conclusion may alleviate some concerns about the possibility of greater problems in initial adjustment to prison for individuals who are facing especially long sentences. On the other hand, as we discussed in the previous chapter, there are likely some deleterious changes in behavior that occur over an extended time in prison. Such changes occurred for all inmates, independently of the amount of time they had left to serve. Thus, the operative variable was the time served, rather than sentence length. Of course, inmates with long sentences will eventually have to serve their time and they will likely be changed as a result. However, the major effects of long sentences occur in serving them, not in having to face them.

10
Predicting Adaptation

Until this point, we have been looking mostly at relationships among different measures that were gathered concurrently, that is, at the same interview. However, our theoretical model says not only that coping and associated appraisals are central to ongoing behavior, but also that they are critical in determining subsequent adaptation. Therefore, one of our primary objectives was to see how well we could predict subsequent behavior and adaptation in prison.

Thus, this chapter will be concerned with the prediction of what happens to individuals over the course of a year or so in prison. The basic strategy was to use measures from the first two interviews, both near the beginning of the term, to predict later adaptation. We used a number of different criteria of adaptation, but each was measured either at the final interview or over the entire period of the study.

Outcome Criteria

Adaptation has many meanings, and it might be measured or indexed in a great variety of ways. We chose five. Two were generated from information in institutional files, and they are categorized very roughly as measures of behavior. The other three criteria were measures of dysphoric, i.e., unpleasant or undesirable, emotional states, as measured at the final interview.

The first type of behavior we used for outcome analyses was subjects' records of disciplinary infractions during the course of the study. We recorded all of the punishments meted out to each subject for reported disciplinary offenses. (In those cases where subjects had been absent from the penitentiary system for periods of longer than 2 weeks, the totals were prorated to estimate amounts for the full period.) In some minor cases, punishments had consisted of warnings only, but we ignored these because they showed the lack of importance of an infraction and because a given individual would be allowed at most one warning.

Table 10.1. Summary of disciplinary and medical data.

Variable	Mean	Range	Percent with none (0)
Disciplinary			
Number of offenses	4.6	0–23	47
Days lost privileges	3.9	0–45	69
Days punitive dissociation	7.8	0–91	73
Days lost remission	7.8	0–69	53
Medical			
Number of initiations	15.1	1–119	0
Number of somatic complaints	8.9	0–85	2
Number of stress-related complaints	4.5	0–54	40
Number of injuries	1.7	0–9	39
Days on meds for stress-related complaints	45.9	0–569	40
Days on psychotropic meds	27.9	0–494	57
Days on other stress meds	18.1	0–329	52

The punishments that were commonly used were, in order of severity, loss of privileges (such as access to entertainment or canteen), punitive dissociation (in ordinary language, solitary confinement), and loss of earned remission (equivalent to an extension of the sentence). Data on each of these measures are summarized in Table 10.1. As can be seen, the majority of inmates were convicted of disciplinary offenses during the time surveyed. Although close to half had no recorded offenses, the range was considerable.

There was also much variance for each of the major types of punishments, although it is interesting that loss of privileges, the least serious sentence, was the least frequently used. This is consistent with our impression that disciplinary charges for small offenses were infrequent, as the bother involved in submitting and processing minor infractions was probably more trouble for guards than these infractions created if ignored. As well, both staff and inmates expressed the opinions that strict adherence to all aspects of regulations created a poor atmosphere and was undesirable. Those offenses that were reported and processed were relatively serious, and therefore the minor punishments such as warnings and removal of privileges were not so frequently used as the heavier punishments of dissociation or loss of remission.

We wanted to derive a single measure to summarize disciplinary history that included both the frequency and seriousness of offenses. Therefore, we formed a composite we called the Discipline Index (DI), formed by adding together normalized values for frequency scores on each of the three types of punishment measures. Thus, the DI is a measure of both the frequency of offenses and the severity of punishments imposed. As such, it should be a reasonable index of difficulties in abiding with institutional rules and routines.

The second index of adjustment that we wanted to survey was medical problems experienced by subjects while they were in prison. To this end, we collected a number of measures of medical symptoms and usage, as summarized in the lower part of Table 10.1. Clearly, subjects had a substantial number of medical problems requiring attention, and the number of initiations, i.e., requests for medical attention, was much higher than one would expect for a group of healthy young males (cf. Heather, 1977).

However, for several reasons the total number of initiations is not a good measure of problems during the term. In many cases the requests for attention were for problems that antedated the beginning of the current prison term. Although we omitted from our count follow-up requests for treatment of a continuing or chronic condition, it was often difficult to judge whether a condition was new. There were also some cases where inmates overused medical facilities, often asking for treatment that was judged not to be medically justified by examining physicians. Although these cases are interesting in themselves, it is hard to see them as measuring real medical problems. Another problem is that, within the system, medical orders were sometimes the only way for inmates to obtain things that do not ordinarily require medical attention on the outside, e.g., dandruff shampoo or special diets. Finally, some inmates sought medical attention in attempts to obtain drugs that could be used for trade or sale within the institution. Again, such cases are not indicative of true health problems.

To arrive at a better measure, the total number of complaints was subdivided into three subcategories: somatic, accidental, and stress-related problems. Injuries attributed to accidents were clearly indicated as such in the medical records. (Of course, this includes some rather peculiar "accidents," such as a surprising number in which inmates claimed to have walked into pipes or tripped on stairways. While we knew that many of these were not truly accidental, it was not possible to differentiate accurately with the available data.)

The category of stress-related complaints included all presenting problems considered to be produced or exacerbated by the effects of stress. This included such things as sleep disturbance, headaches, or gastrointestinal distress, unless there was a contradictory diagnosis, such as the presence of a disease or infectious process. Chronic conditions were classed as general somatic problems if they had begun before the start of the term, even though they might have had stress-related origins, except if they became acutely worse during the study. The somatic category was otherwise generally defined by exclusion, i.e., problems that were attributable to causes other than stress or accidents.

As can be seen from Table 10.1, stress-related problems comprised about 30% of the total, and it was these that were of particular interest for our study. We would expect that failures to cope adequately with situations might produce some physiological strain; over time, this pressure would lead to stress-related medical symptomatology. Therefore, stress-related symptoms were the medical occurrences of most interest for us.

As our actual Medical Index (MI) we used the number of days on which a subject had received medication for stress-related complaints. This measure has some advantage over the number of complaints, in that it does not include complaints that were judged to be medically unjustified or trivial by qualified medical practicioners. Also, since prescriptions for most medications are strictly regulated in the system and must be renewed regularly, long courses of treatment should be associated only with persistent or serious problems. As with the DI, the MI was corrected for extended absences from the penitentiary system.

To give further detail, the total of medications received can be further divided according to the actual drugs chosen, and, as Table 10.1 shows, about 60% were psychotropic drugs including major and minor tranquilizers. The remainder were a variety of specifics for stress-related complaints, mostly those that are classically considered as psychosomatic.

The final three outcome criteria were all measures of emotional state. Depression and anxiety are the most common results of an inability to handle stressful events. The Beck Depression Index (BDI) and the Spielberger State Anxiety Index (STAI) had been administered at each interview because of their established validity and widespread clinical use. We used scores at the final interview as our measures of final state.

We also wanted to measure anger because it is another likely result of coping problems, and because we knew that it is an especially common problem among inmates. Unfortunately, we could not find a measure that had been previously validated and was generally accepted. Therefore, we used a simple measure that had been obtained from our questionnaires: the score on the anger subset of the Mood Adjective Checklist. This score is simply the number of anger-related adjectives that a subject indicated as descriptive of his current feelings. In the absence of a better measure, we chose it as a convenient Anger Index (AI).

Because they were taken from files, the DI and MI could be calculated for almost all subjects, even those who were not available for the third interview. However, the emotional indices depended on completion of the interview, so the number of subjects for whom they were available was reduced to just under 100.

Core Variables and Simple Correlations

We wanted to relate each outcome criterion to measures taken early in the term. However, there were so many measures from the first two interviews that it would have been tedious, impractical, and statistically undesirable to use them all. Therefore, we chose for our analyses an abbreviated set of core variables covering a number of different areas.

To represent coping and associated behaviors we chose measures that had been prominent in the patterns of behavior described in the previous several chapters. For example, these included measures of socialization, planning of time, and past coping difficulties, as well as the efficacy of coping in prison. We also included several measures of cognitions and appraisals in order to have information about subjects' current thinking patterns and experiences, because these are also important in the coping process. As a third set we included a variety of socioeconomic and personal background factors, from a measure of family intactness in childhood (family type) to the number of criminal convictions. Finally, to confirm the lack of important effects seen in the previous chapter, we added sentence length and the level of confinement to the set.

The final set for the analyses in this chapter consisted of 24 variables, most taken at the first interview. However, the Prison Problems Scale had not been administered until the second interview, and to allow it to correspond to other measures of related behavior in the same time period, measures of coping, total problems, and thoughts of the past and future were also taken from the second interview.

In the first set of analyses, we computed correlations between each of the set of 24 measures and the 5 outcome criteria, with the results shown in Table 10.2. Given the sheer number of different correlations represented, not much can be said about the pattern. It is obvious that there is much variation in the importance of the relationships, both across predictor variables and criteria.

It can also be seen that there is a great deal of specificity, such that each criterion is related to a different set of variables, i.e., different outcomes are differently determined. In general, it appears that background factors are less predictive than the others. Comparing across outcome criteria, the DI was significantly related to 14 of the 24 predictors, several more than any of the others.

If we consider specific correlations, one important result to notice is that some variables are significantly related to several different criteria, but in opposite directions. For example, the more friends a subject had, the less likely he was to suffer from each of the dysphoric emotions, but the more disciplinary offenses he was likely to acquire. Thinking about the future was associated with more stress-related physical symptoms over the term, but less anxiety at the end. Attempts by subjects to control their thoughts predicted slightly lower disciplinary and medical rates but higher anxiety.

From these results it appears that there may not be such a thing as a single optimal set of responses for coping with situations in prison. Given that stressful situations occur, an inmate has the choice of dealing with them in ways that direct the damage, but it may sometimes be impossible to avoid all deleterious consequences. Of course, the most successful ways of coping result in long-term solutions that remove problems, and in such cases there may be no negative consequences. However, as we have discussed before, many of the problems faced by prisoners are almost inevitable results of imprisonment, e.g., missing loved ones. In such cases, the numbers in Table 10.2 show that a coping strategy that averts one possible

TABLE 10.2. Correlations of major variables with outcome measures.

Predictor variables	Outcome variables				
	Discipline	Medical	Depression	Anxiety	Anger
Background					
Sentence length	.08	−.00	−.02	.10	−.04
Social class	−.27**	−.21*	−.23*	−.12	−.11
Family type	−.28**	.07	−.07	−.08	−.10
School level	−.12	−.15*	−.19*	−.09	−.02
Marital status	−.10	.05	.07	.10	−.12
Age	−.27**	−.03	.10	.04	−.24*
Nbr. convictions	.22**	.14	.15	.12	.22*
Custody level	.19*	−.00	.20*	.02	−.11
General coping					
Alcohol abuse	.42***	.27**	.16	.10	.25**
Suicide attempts	.19*	.34***	.11	.12	.10
Efficacy	−.29**	−.18*	.01	−.04	.19*
Specific behavior and coping					
How socialize	.12	−.08	−.10	−.06	−.01
Nbr friends	.18*	.10	−.26**	−.32**	−.21*
Cell time	−.07	−.12	−.19*	.03	−.12
Nbr letters	−.01	−.09	−.10	−.03	−.14
Plan or day × day	−.23**	−.10	−.15	.00	−.03
Type of plans	−.17*	−.29***	−.19*	−.17	−.08
Control thoughts?	−.21*	−.17*	−.00	.23*	−.13
Future thoughts	.14	.21*	−.16	−.36***	−.13
Past thoughts	.03	.06	−.15	−.30**	−.37***
Appraisals					
Prison problems	.32***	.12	.48***	.54***	.39***
Total problems	.35***	.37***	.54***	.47***	.30*
I–E scale	−.11	−.12	−.36***	−.23*	−.20*
Freq boredom	−.00	.14	.18*	.31**	.36***

*$p<.05$
**$p<.01$
***$p<.001$

unpleasant outcome may also increase the likelihood of a different undesirable outcome.

On one level, this implies that there is a tradeoff in behavior. Actions that mitigate the effects of problem situations in one direction may aggravate them in another. One must choose one's objective in order to specify the best way of reaching it, and there may be some clash between objectives. Moreover, every objective implies a choice: one must sometimes sail a narrow behavioral course between a Scylla and Charybdis of maladaptive consequences.

If we generalize speculatively, we might say that such a situation reflects the limitations of adaptation in everyday life. Every benefit has its costs, and the roads we choose to follow determine the potholes into which we will fall. Psychological survival comes at the cost of some inevitable difficulties. Of course, the better one is able to cope, the easier may be the path overall, but there is no strategy that does not have its failings somewhere. The conflicts between outcomes seen in our data indicate that perfect coping is not attainable.

On a theoretical level, we are led to call into question any unitary notions of stress and adaptation. Discussions of adaptation must specify the criterion more clearly and more specifically than in the past. In the end, it may be that adaptation can be defined only in terms of the relationship between specific behaviors and particular outcomes. Otherwise, a given behavior might appear to be both adaptive and maladaptive, depending on one's choice of criterion. It is all too easy to look at a single criterion of maladaptive behavior, in the expectation that other measures will work similarly. The results of comparing predictors of several different concurrent criteria of adaptation show the fallacy of such assumptions.

Predictive Analyses

Although some important features stand out, as a whole the pattern of correlations in Table 10.2 is too complex to assimilate. It is also difficult to interpret statistically, as one does not know how individual correlations add together. For example, if two related measures each correlate with a given criterion, it may show two independent sources of determination or just that the two measures are redundant. One needs to use more comprehensive analyses to deal with these problems.

Thus, in order to see better the pattern of determinants for each criterion, we performed a set of regression analyses. Briefly, this statistical technique generates an equation that uses a combination of variables to predict an outcome measure. There are a variety of regression procedures, but we calculated first a set of stepwise analyses in which the entire set of 23 predictors (sentence length was now dropped because it was so clearly irrelevant) was allowed to enter the equation for each criterion. The computational algorithm for this type of analysis enters variables into the equation in the order of their power to predict the outcome, and stops when additional variables would make no significant additions to prediction of the criterion.

The results may be seen in Table 10.3, which shows the predictors entering into the equations for each outcome measure, and the order of their entry. Overall, the pattern of results confirms and strengthens what was visible from the simple correlational analyses.

Looking first at the results of all five analyses together, we can see that there is some variation among measures in the final proportion of variance accounted for (r^2), that is, how well they were predicted by the measures we used. However, in general the final level of prediction was quite good

TABLE 10.3. Summaries of regression analyses with outcome measures.

Predictor variables	Outcome variables				
	Discipline	Medical	Depression	Anxiety	Anger
Background					
Social class					
Family type	6				
School level					
Marital status					
Age	4		4		4
Nbr. convictions					6
Custody level	7		5		
General Coping					
Alcohol abuse	1				
Suicide attempts		1			
Efficacy	8				
Specific behavior and coping					
How socialize		6	7		
Nbr friends	3	7			
Cell time		3	6		
Nbr letters			8		5
Plan or day × day	5				
Type of plans		2		3	
Control thoughts?				4	
Future thoughts		5		2	
Past thoughts					2
Appraisals					
Prison problems	2		1	1	1
Total problems		4	2	5	
I–E scale			3	7	7
Freq boredom				6	3
Final r	.654	.531	.606	.652	.611
Final r²	.428	.282	.368	.424	.374
Final r² (adj)	.390	.241	.327	.392	.338

considering the limitations in the outcome indices themselves. The file data on which the first two measures were based were sometimes incomplete or unclear, and the reliabilities of the emotional measures were somewhat imperfect, so the attained levels probably represent a high proportion of the reliable variance for most of the criteria.

Thus, we conclude that some important measures of adaptation can be predicted by a coping analysis. It should be stressed that our predictive measures were taken at least a year in advance of the outcome measures; that is, we were truly predicting those outcomes. Equally important is the fact that the measures used were chosen for theoretical reasons rather than just because they were useful as predictors.

Our analyses do have some similarity to those in previous studies, especially some of those predicting recidivism (e.g., Hoffman, 1983; Nuffield,

1982). However, previous analyses have not fulfilled the conditions we imposed. For example, the set of variables that have been identified as predictors of recidivism are actuarial in nature, with predictors gathered together only because as a group they happen to allow some level of prediction. In these cases, the rationale for the selection of predictors is entirely empirical; no matter how impressive the results, they are of very limited use in building or assessing an understanding of the causal networks that determine an outcome. This is in contrast to our own approach, in which the predictor variables were almost all chosen to represent aspects of the theoretical model we have been testing, and where the same set of predictors was used for five different criteria.

Indeed, the analyses reported here are not individually the most powerful predictors that we could generate for our respective criterion measures. In exploring the data we performed a number of other analyses, and we found that we could substantially increase the proportions of explained variance over those shown here by varying (and especially by enlarging) the set of predictor variables. In general, we could come close to doubling the proportion of predicted variance for each of the criteria. However, such analyses are not as theoretically relevant as those we chose to include. Our design uniquely allows us to evaluate how well a theoretically justified set of measures can predict subsequent adaptation. Any other analyses are much less powerful for an understanding of behavior, regardless of the figures.

If we look at the results of Table 10.3 in greater detail, we can see that the variables entering into the regression were different for each criterion, i.e., the things that predict adaptation are not the same for all aspects of adaptation. These results are another demonstration that different measures of adjustment do not work in the same way. The factors determining such things as disciplinary problems and depression, during the same period and under the same environmental and individual circumstances, are not the same.

Thus, the present pattern of results shows that the predictors of different criteria of adaptation in the same environment vary widely. Given this variation, we might ask whether the obtained results are each characteristic of the chosen criteria, or whether they are idiosyncratic results determined by the unique combinations of criteria, environment, and our set of subjects. For example, would the same set of variables predict a given criterion as successfully as here if we were to use different subjects or different environments?

While these are questions that must be answered empirically, we can predict from our theoretical position that a replication with different subjects should yield essentially the same results, for we have generally assumed that there is little that is unique among prison inmates other than the facts of their offenses and imprisonment. We would probably also say much the same thing about the results of testing the model in different environments. Except where a situation contains unique elements, we would expect that the determinants of a given aspect of adaptation would be much the same everywhere. Thus, we would expect that the determinants of depression in a population of university undergraduates would be much like those in our analysis for prison inmates, or that anxiety among carpenters could be predicted by the same measures useful for prisoners. Of course, this does not mean that a given individual would adapt the same in different situations, and it certainly does not say that the average adaptation on any given criterion would be the same across situations. Rather, we assume that the same sorts of processes are active in almost any normal environment, regardless of its features.

Although we have no data that bear directly on these questions, we can cite some indirect evidence indicating the similarity of determinants across environments. For example, the factors predictive of the number of disciplinary offenses in prison are quite similar to those correlated with the number of criminal offenses committed outside of prison by our subjects, and also with the variables predicting recidivism in some actuarial studies like those cited earlier. Except for our use of coping measures and the emphasis on specific behaviors, the set of measures predictive of DI in Tables 10.2 or 10.3 could be mistaken for yet one more recidivism prediction table. Thus, it seems that within limits the same measures might predict misconduct or antisocial behavior across a variety of situations.

If we return to comparing the sets of predictors for each criterion, we can see some other results of interest. In particular, it appears that background factors as a whole are generally not very prominent in the regression equations. Age appeared in the sets for 3 of the 5 criteria, but as the fourth variable each time, and among the others only the custody level of the institution to which a subject was originally assigned appeared twice. Three of the 7 included background variables did not appear at all.

In contrast, coping and appraisal factors were relatively more powerful as predictors, appearing on the average about twice as frequently as the background variables. Interestingly, the behavioral criteria, DI and MI, were most closely linked with measures of overt behavior, while cognitive appraisals were very important for predicting each of the three emotional states.

To provide a summary and comparison of the influence of each type of measure, we performed an additional set of regression analyses. In these, the same variables as before were entered. However, they were entered at different times, in four groups, and the entire set was entered rather than just those selected as most powerful by the algorithm employed by the analysis. Background measures were entered first, followed by generalized coping measures, then specific current behaviors, and finally the measures of problem appraisals and generalized cognitions.

This technique is a fairly direct way of comparing the predictive power of the different sets of variables. It determines whether together the variables

TABLE 10.4. Significance of change in outcome variance produced by each set of predictor variables.

Predictor set	Outcome variables				
	Discipline	Medical	Depression	Anxiety	Anger
Background	***	—	—	—	—
Coping general	***	***	—	—	—
Current behavior	—	*	**	***	***
Appraisals	**	—	***	***	**
Final r	.69	.59	.67	.69	.64
Final r^2	.48	.35	.45	.48	.41

$*p<.05$
$**p<.01$
$***p<.001$

in each set add significantly to the power of the regression equation to explain the variance in the criterion. If there is predictive power that is duplicated in two predictors, it will be attributed to the one that is allowed to enter the equation first, so the analyses give more chance to see effects from the variables entered earlier. Thus, it can be seen that in comparing background and coping-process factors we decided to favor the former.

The results, shown in Table 10.4, indicate even better than the previous analyses how the different types of predictors are related to each of the outcome measures. As can be seen, the set of background factors was significantly predictive only for the disciplinary history, in spite of its statistical advantage. In contrast, the general coping set adds significantly to prediction for the two behavioral criteria, and each of the other two sets makes significant contributions for four of the five outcomes. Thus, coping and appraisal measures go far beyond background factors in predicting subsequent outcomes. If one considers these analyses to be a fair comparison of the usefulness of the different types of factors, then they demonstrate that coping theory allows a considerable advance in predictive and explanatory power beyond that possible with previous models.

Comparing across outcome criteria, we can again see some differences. For example, the DI seems to be more widely determined than the other criteria, with significant contributions from three of the four sets. In contrast, each of the other criteria is related to only two types of measures. Our index of medical symptoms is best predicted by coping-related measures, both general and specific. All three of the emotional criteria show contributions only from current behaviors and cognitive appraisals, reinforcing our previous conclusions that emotional states are more closely linked to thoughts and cognitions than to anything else.

This is as one might expect, since specific activities ought to be influential in determining overt behavior, while emotions are largely under the control of specific thoughts and generalized ways of interpreting events. The great bulk of recent theorizing has assumed that emotional responses are mediated by cognitions. For example, depression has been linked with specific cognitive antecedents (Beck, 1976). While some previous evidence, especially that of Beck and his colleagues, has shown differences in cognitions between depressed and nondepressed individuals, there has been little in the way of predictive demonstrations. The present study provides such evidence, showing that depression can indeed be predicted from expectations, attributions, and appraisals.

Some Consequences

From the evidence in this chapter, we conclude that the approach we have taken does allow us to predict something about subsequent behavior and adaptation in prison. The analyses presented here show that an individual's adjustment or maladjustment after a year in prison is at least predictable from his initial behavior in the institution, and imply further that the behaviors and cognitions underlying our predictor variables actually determine the subsequent adaptation. Still, while the level of prediction may be somewhat better than that of previous theoretical models, it is far from perfect, and there is room for substantial improvement. We believe that the most likely path to better prediction is in refinements to the coping theory or its replacement with another similar interactionist model.

We had expected many of the results visible in the various regression analyses, and they are consistent with the pattern of results presented in previous chapters. The difference in this chapter is in the emphasis on prediction rather than just correlations among concomitant measures. The power of any theory can be best assessed in its predictive ability; the evidence included here shows that there are at least some elements of the present approach that are of important value.

At the same time, if our results here are not surprising to us theoretically, they do emphasize again the gap between empirical knowledge and current practice in corrections. In several respects, we can see that our results and conclusions are in contrast with common contemporary practices.

For example, we can return to the issue of the treatment of long-term offenders raised in the previous chapter. In conversations we were told that current policies were based on the expectation that people who had committed serious and violent crimes on the outside were those who were likely to do the same inside prison. However, our data on adaptation show how mistaken this assumption is. Sentence length does not predict any important measure of adaptation in prison, from disciplinary history to depression. In using it as the basis for assignment, correctional officials ensure that future disruptions will be spread more or less randomly throughout the system.

Such mistakes are not only unjust to prisoners, but they also create some difficulties for management of inmate behavior by prison authorities. For example, under the policy of assigning offenders to institutions on the basis of sentence length, many inmates who do not need close supervision are assigned to maximum-security institutions, thus using resources unnecessarily. Conversely, the same policy allows other inmates to create disciplinary problems in lower-security institutions before they can be transferred out, because the risks they present were not anticipated. Thus, the system pays a price for ignorance, and the lack of ability to predict inmates' behavior interferes with good institutional management.

This problem is a good example of how policies based on inadequate behavioral assumptions are contrary to the interests of all parties in the institutions. However, it is not the only case where current practice differs sharply from the implications of our data. Another instance can be seen in the role of institutional staff in fostering inmate social networks. As can be seen from the data, inmates' involvement in socialization with other prisoners is positively correlated with the incidence of disciplinary problems. Yet it was common in the system for staff to approve of such networks as promoters of stability and to encourage participation by individual inmates as a sign of adjustment to the prison.

Other similar cases in the data are readily apparent. For now, the examples above are sufficient to make it clear that in many ways contemporary prisons are designed on the basis of erroneous or outdated behavioral assumptions.

The reasons for this are probably mostly based in the historical development of our present institutions, but there is certainly great resistance to change. In any institution or system of institutions, procedures become enshrined by long usage, and are afterwards supported by such resistance to change. However, in the case of prisons, policies and procedures are also reinforced by much mythology about behavior that is not consonant with reality.

We believe that the assumptions behind policies should be subject to empirical tests. Institutional rules and procedures should be made consonant with behavior in the prison as it actually occurs, rather than with preconceptions and assumptions. Our data demonstrate how inmates' behavior in prison can be predicted; methods similar to ours can be used more widely to determine the details of inmates' behavior. If this were done, we believe that institutional rules and procedures could be changed for the betterment of both inmates and institutions. The perpetuation of policies based on ignorance serves neither.

11
Conclusions: What Prisons Do and Don't Do

From all of the previous parts of this monograph, one can see how individual ways of reacting to situations combine with external conditions to produce the observable varieties of everyday behavior. We have been able to generate a coherent behavioral picture of the lives of criminal offenders, both outside and inside prison, and we can even connect that pricture to their offenses. In the previous chapter we showed how a coping analysis can be used to predict subsequent adaptation, and it is clear that the present approach works much better than those limited to traditional sorts of background and historical measures. Thus, we find evidence for the claim that the determination of behavior lies in the interaction of external and internal factors.

It should be obvious that our results have substantial implications for both theory and practice related to the treatment of criminal offenders. On one level, we are in a position to make a number of concrete suggestions about the functioning of contemporary prisons. If we are asked how our data can be used to direct improvements in the penal system, many areas become apparent. Most of these have already been indicated in previous chapters. For example, we have discussed at some length how our analyses of the predictors of adaptation can be used to provide better policies for assigning inmates to institutions. Another area is the timing of treatment programs within a prison term.

These are only a few examples of how current prison practices seem to be based on unfounded assumptions about inmates' behavior. They are certainly not isolated or unique. From the first dealings of an inmate with the correctional system, it is obvious that decisions are made on the basis of incorrect assumptions or incomplete information, and when we compare actual operations of the system to the implications from our findings we can easily find many other places where changes can be recommended.

However, most of these areas where our data relate to current practice have already been indicated and discussed in previous chapters, and there is no need to reiterate the arguments here. Instead, in this discussion we will return to the larger issues of the general effects of imprisonment that were considered in chapter 1.

As we have stressed, conditions in prison are very different from those on the outside. Imprisonment by its nature requires that inmates will live apart from their families, live together in groups that would not otherwise exist, and be seriously constrained in their choices. As a result, the prison world is socially and psychologically artificial. One of our primary objectives in undertaking this study was to further our understanding of what prisons do to the imprisoned. In this chapter, we will develop our conclusions about the general effects of imprisonment.

What Prisons Do *Not* Do: The Breaking Ground

In considering all of the possible effects of imprisonment, it is clear that a great many claims that have been made in the past are not supported by the evidence in this study. It is appropriate to consider these negative findings first: This section is concerned with claims or hypotheses about the effects of imprisonment that we could not substantiate.

Among the claims about the effects of imprisonment, there are two sorts of harmful or injurious effects that are often cited, and both may be seen in the litany of hypothesized effects presented in chapter 1. The first is that prison leads to a high frequency of deterioration among prisoners. The form of this hypothesized damage varies, but it usually includes reductions in intellectual abilities, loss of capacities to deal with life on the outside, or even generalized and permanent emotional harm. Usually, the damage is linked to the lack of stimulation and monotony in prison, along with the lack of choices and the dependency imposed on inmates.

While there are thus many varied claims about prison-induced deterioration, previous evidence has been inconclusive. If we generalize, we can say that there are single-case reports purporting to show serious emotional, intellectual, or social impairment resulting from imprisonment, but more controlled studies are sparse and fail to show any general deteriorative effects. As a longitudinal study with a substantial sample size, the present investigation can therefore provide some critical data about generalized deterioration in prison, at least for terms on the order of a year or two.

Our data on emotional states indicate that there are severe problems at the beginning of a prison term for many inmates. However, for most the disturbance is fortunately evanescent, and over the course of time it seems to dissipate. The evident distress is serious, and more resources should be made available for its treatment than are currently available in most penal institutions: One cannot lightly dismiss emotional disturbances for the reason that they will last only a year or so. However, at the same time we can say that in general imprisonment does not produce much in the way of generalized or lasting dysphoric emotional disturbance.

This allows us to reinterpret previous claims, for we can see that the effect one finds will depend on the time of measurement. Accounts of the initial experience of imprisonment are bound to reflect the widespread depression and anxiety we were able to measure, but descriptions or measurements done later in a term will show more the dulling of sensations attributable to sameness and routine. Some of the apparent conflict in previous reports can be resolved with this in mind.

The data in this study are also congruent with the results of other recent systematic studies of the effects of imprisonment, as reviewed in the introductory chapter. We went somewhat beyond previous studies with use of a longitudinal design, and also with measurements starting near the beginning of subjects' terms in prison. We also surveyed behavior and adaptation in a number of areas that had not previously been assessed. Given the differences in methodology, the similarity of results seems all the more significant. In summary, we may say that, taken together with previous results, our data indicate that general deterioration does not occur.

If the prediction of deteriorative effects is based on the deprivations in prisons, expectations of the occurrence of the second category of harmful effects come from observations that there are some aspects of prison life that are unique to that environment. It is assumed that the presence of such elements leads to maladaptive changes that will persist and cause problems after release. We examined several predictions of models assuming that offenders acquire maladaptive habits in prison, and in each case the predictions were contradicted by the data. For example, there was no suggestion of any substantial changes in either specific ways of coping or in generalized coping ability. Indeed, there were very few systematic changes over time for overt behaviors of any sort.

There is every reason to expect that we would have seen the development of maladaptive prison behaviors if they had occurred, for our longitudinal design was quite sensitive to changes within a term. Certainly, our 16-month period of measurement allowed ample time for changes to develop and become visible. Moreover, we could see no special effects in first-time offenders, who would have been expected to show the most change.

We did find that inmates with greater amounts of previous prison experience were worse in coping with problems in their lives. However, there was no sign of any change in this pattern over the course of the term; rather, prisoners who coped well at the beginning of their terms mostly coped well later. The average amount of time in prison previous to the index sentence was, fortuitously, about the same as the interval covered by our set of interviews. From this, one would need to argue that any maladaptive learning that occurs in prison must develop within a time no longer than our subjects had served previously, and, therefore, that such effects would be visible across interviews. However, the results did not support this supposition, so the initial differences are best interpreted as a statistical fallout from a filtering process in which habitual offenders are differentiated from others. That is, we expect that the worst copers among released prisoners are those most likely to commit new offenses and return to prison, and eventually the poorest copers among the population of offenders will be those with the longest criminal records.

We would not deny that some men suffer deterioration of various types in prison, and we feel sure that if we looked long and hard enough we would find some changes that are common across prisoners. Yet, such changes would be neither surprising nor unusual, for people change throughout their lives, and aging alone does great damage to many abilities in all of us. It should not be assumed that such effects would be the results of imprisonment. Many writers of single-case or autobiographical studies (and unfortunately even some well-known investigators) have committed the simple logical error of assuming that any change that develops *while* a man is in prison must have occurred *because* he is in prison ("post hoc, ergo propter hoc").

Rather, what must be shown is a risk of a particular type of deterioration that is higher than might have been expected without imprisonment. Given the prior problems that our data show among our subjects, from suicide attempts to an extremely high amount of alcohol consumption, it would be remarkable if we did not see some physical and intellectual deterioration. The general lack of such systematic changes in our data is therefore a bit surprising, although the focus of this investigation was not on physical or intellectual functioning. Thus, we can see no evidence that maladaptive ways of reacting are acquired in prison.

Even more, it does not appear that imprisonment has much of an effect on prisoners' general ways of thinking about, or reacting to, situations and circumstances. From the patterns visible in our results, we can see that imprisonment had only a transitory effect on most aspects of our subjects' ways of living. After the initial disruption, in many ways we could see the reassertion of their initial ways of reacting to events. For example, the aimless unplanned lifestyle on the outside was interrupted at the beginning by some efforts at planning and interest in self-improvement, but after a while most of the impetus for change had evaporated in the winds of drifting time. We conclude that most of the effects of prison on individuals are impermanent and situational. From this we would predict that once the physical constraints of prison on behavior are removed, most men will return to some approximation of their behavior before imprisonment, without any greatly increased risk of permanent damage or deterioration.

The claim that substantial damage does not occur should not be taken as an endorsement of the use of imprisonment. For one thing, despite the general improvement over time, our data show that some individuals continued to be disturbed even well into their terms. Some of this may be the result of a deliberate self-imposed psychological isolation such as may be indicated by some of the changes we observed at our final interview, but there is a need for further research to identify these individuals and what makes them react differently, so that help can be arranged.

In addition, it should be apparent that our conclusions are based on intervals equivalent to prison terms of short to intermediate length. Without follow-up of longer duration we can say little about the effects of very long sentences. Still, we expect that most men would show impairment of certain sorts after very long stretches of time in prison.

In our rapidly changing world, there is bound to be some culture shock for inmates released after several years of isolation from major ongoing changes. For example, we have heard stories from inmates who were unable to function in stores because they had been in prison during the worst of the inflationary cycle in the 70s and could not estimate changed prices of things after their release; others had trouble in making legal withdrawals from banks because computerization had changed the procedures while they were in prison. Problems like these are far from unique in our society, and the difficulties that we can expect released long-term inmates to experience are probably very similar to those of immigrants in a new culture. These problems are likely only temporary and they can be overcome with some persistence and experience. Still, there is much about long-term acculturation that we do not know, so even with the help of the immigrant analogy we can reach no informed conclusion about possible permanent effects of very long terms in prison.

Nevertheless, in spite of the reservations outlined above, we conclude that prisons do not produce permanent harm to the psychological well-being of inmates. While we feel that this conclusion is reasonably justified by the data, in some ways it is paradoxical. Although we have tried to avoid lurid descriptions of suffering and brutality in our depiction of prison conditions, we are well aware of the unpleasantness of prison life. Why then does imprisonment not permanently damage people?

The best answer we can provide relates to the centrality of coping in our understanding of adaptation. Even if prisoners are in general relatively poor in coping with everyday events, they do manage to survive in the hostile situations that prisons present. Indeed, as we have discussed in chapter 7, the ways that offenders react to situations are often more adaptive in prisons than on the outside. Prisoners are often perverse in their adaptations, but they provide good examples of the remarkable behavioral adaptability of human beings, and they manage to find ways of coping that allow them to remain mostly unchanged and undamaged. However, on the whole it must be said that this survival intact does not occur because of the conditions that prisons present, but in spite of them.

What Prisons *Do*: The Deep Freeze

We have concluded that the attribution of disastrous effects to imprisonment is one of the many myths common in the criminological literature. It should be remembered that evidence presented earlier in chapter 7 had led us to a similar argument. Thus, although our conclusions are essentially negative, they are broadly based on a number of internally consistent sources of evidence.

Still, the failure to find evidence of generalized or long-lasting damage can provide only very scant support for the widespread use of imprisonment. The great costs of prisons, both financial and psychological, demand that they provide some substantial positive benefits as well. If we except the possible uses of prisons to satisfy motives of vengeance or unthinking retribution, then the benefits should be visible in the ways that prisons change and improve the behavior of inmates to make them less likely to commit new offenses.

Our data provide some evidence about the occurrence of such positive changes. We would have expected to see some effects in various places in our data. Most especially, in the comparisons of repeated measures across interviews we should have seen changes that might benefit inmates' behavior after release

Given our expectations about the role of coping responses in the genesis of adaptive or maladaptive behaviors, the most critical changes would have been improvements in coping over the course of imprisonment. However, the data actually showed very little change in coping behavior over time. There was a very small increase in measured efficacy across interviews, but this would not be enough to effect much of a change in adaptation. In terms of specific types of coping responses, the only trends visible were increases by some inmates in the use of a few modalities that are particularly useful in dealing with the sort of insoluble problems that imprisonment presents. Thus, we have little reason to say that prisons improve coping or that there is any real prospect for better coping by inmates after release.

We also see little or no evidence for positive changes in other areas of behavior. For example, we have hypothesized that the commission of criminal offenses on the outside is linked to an unstructured loose lifestyle, with little consideration of any time period outside the immediate present. This was not changed in prison, for the institutions allowed or even encouraged the same lifestyle.

In attempting to find other possible changes in inmates that might be considered benefits of their time in prison, we looked at all of the other measures that were measured repeatedly in our study. As discussed earlier, we did not find significant changes in any of the important measures of ongoing behavior. Neither were there major visible changes in cognitions, thoughts, or attitudes, whether restricted to those about prison or widened to those about life in general.

Thus, we can see little evidence that prisons promote positive changes in inmates. As they had done on the outside, most of the inmates in this study followed a path of least resistance, and they focused on the fine line of present time passing. They found it easier to serve time, as they were sentenced to do, by passing through it, rather than using it.

An apparent exception to the above generalization is seen in the set of measures that led us to write in chapter 6 of a window of opportunity. However, this did not last long, and after a few months most inmates had fallen back to following the demands of the immediate environment and to relying on routine to get through their days. If there are opportunities for permanent change in prison, they can hardly be said to represent a positive effect of imprisonment, for the system does not capitalize on them. This is most unfortunate: inmates may experience the pains of imprisonment, but any consequent gains do not seem to materialize.

To summarize, we would argue that our data show very little positive behavioral change in prison, just as earlier we could see little evidence for generalized negative effects. What then are the effects of imprisonment? On one level, we can say that prison is a unique environment, but one within the range of ordinary human experience, so its effects are as varied as those of any major life change on a disparate group of individuals. Some men sink into depression and hopelessness, while others feel comfortable, contented, or even happy. From our results we can say that most fall somewhere in between, coping day by day and minute by minute, and surviving intact and more or less unchanged.

This is all consistent with our arguments about the limited effect of environmental conditions alone on behavior. If individual ways of reacting must always be factored into the results of external circumstances, so the effects of prisons will vary across individuals. Compared to the power of the interaction between events and individual responses, imprisonment in itself is not sufficient to produce any consistent changes in behavior, at least not in any area that we and other systematic researchers have surveyed.

Of course, this does not mean that prisons do not have some power to impose uniformity on ongoing behavior. While in prison, the force of regulations and conditions is a very powerful determinant of behavior. Although the control of the environment is far from total, in essential areas prisoners are forced to conform or suffer losses. Moreover, as the prison environment is less varied than conditions on the outside, so is the behavior of inmates more uniform.

However, these constraints are largely on rather peripheral aspects of external behavior. What we observe is that more central aspects, such as general cognitions, remain unchanged, at least over the course of a year or so in prison. Even more important, the patterns of behavior resulting from the constraints of imprisonment do not reflect any real learning process, and therefore they are bound to last no longer than the constraints that induce them. The reasons for this can be seen from considering something of what we know about the psychology of learning.

To begin with, we can see that the alterations in behavior that occur during imprisonment are immediate effects of the environment, as shown in chapter 6, and they require no active accommodation on the part of prisoners. The inmate does not have to learn to awaken early; unless he is deaf, he will be unable to sleep through the morning noise in an institution. He does not have to learn to organize his time, for his schedule is imposed by administrative fiat. In short, when men are imprisoned their behavioral patterns change almost immediately to fit the new environment, and, as shown before, there is a general lack of further changes later in the term.

Thus, the changes in behavior imposed by imprisonment are passively imposed, and not the results of any learning process. Because of this, we would expect any changes to disappear upon release. While behavior may change temporarily in response to environmental demands, in the absence of any mechanism to maintain them the new behaviors will disappear as soon as they are no longer induced by the environment. Habits are changed by reinforcements and contingencies, not by practice.

The necessary conditions for permanent behavioral change are not present in prison. Given the rule of bureaucracy, while a man is in prison the contingencies between his behavior and the outcomes he receives are minimal. Punishments for some proscribed behaviors may possibly reduce rates of occurrence, but even these contingencies are uncertainly and inconsistently applied. Even more important is an almost complete lack of rewards for desirable behaviors. With the organization of most contemporary prisons, it is inevitable that the mechanisms of learning will not be effectively evoked to produce any lasting behavioral change. As a generalization, we might say that prison affects men strongly, but in the long run it changes them hardly at all.

Thus, if we see no evidence for permanent behavioral change in our subjects, such a result is predictable from what we know about behavioral processes in general. By extension, we can also see why prisons fail to change behavior in the outside world by inmates who have been released from prison. In the end, individuals who enter prison with inadequate behavioral repertoires or maladaptive modes of coping are bound to leave with the same (lack of) capabilities. While men are in prison their outside behavior patterns remain, in effect, frozen in time. Indeed, we can characterize imprisonment as the behavioral equivalent of a deep freeze, in which the outside behavior of inmates is stored until their release.

We believe that this description best summarizes the entire pattern of results from our study. Although the deep freeze notion is not apodictic, it is an effective heuristic, and using it we can begin to see more clearly why prisons fail.

Amid the general lack of evidence for the learning of new behaviors in prison, the lack of change in coping stands out for us. Ordinarily, we expect that learning to cope well involves the action of experience and environmental feedback, interacting with native abilities and response propensities. On the basis of our data we would argue that most offenders have deficiencies somewhere in this process, and that they arrive in prison with poor coping ability. Imprisonment then deprives them of experience with the normal environment, and thus limits their further experience with conditions that they must deal with on the outside. Most of us learn to cope better through accumulated experience, but prisoners are deprived of much of that experience. As a result, they do not learn to cope satisfactorily with conditions in the outside world.

Thus, as well as having his behavior frozen in its original pattern, the prisoner is frozen developmentally. This might explain why the behavior of habitual offenders resembles that of adolescents in many ways, e.g., in the heavy dependence on peer groups, emphasis on physical dominance, and generally impulsive behavioral style. It also follows that imprisonment at an early age will have more effect on subsequent behavior than at a later time. Finally, from this analysis we can predict (or postdict, in the present case) that those who have spent the most time in prison will cope most poorly when they are on the outside. And according to the coping–criminality hypothesis this would then lead them to commit new offenses, resulting in their return to prison, and a return to the cycle, ad infinitum.

We are thus led to a pessimistic appraisal of the possibilities in the present system. The notion of the deep freeze leads us to expect that for each inmate there is a point where further imprisonment may trap him into a cycle of regular recidivism. If prisons do not actively interfere with good coping or adaptive behavior, neither do they promote their development.

These conclusions derive from our observations about the lack of behavioral changes during a prison term. However, they are not solely dependent on those data or on the arguments above about the (lack of) behavioral contingencies and learning in prison.

Even if prisoners did learn new and better ways of coping while they were in prison, they would still be unlikely to improve their behavior on the outside, for we know from the experimental literature that learning is situation-specific. This is because the evocation of a behavior is strongly linked to the presence of stimuli that were present when that behavior was learned. Many of us are familiar with the example of the housecat jumping on the forbidden kitchen table as soon as we—the set of controlling stimuli—leave the room.

Students of the psychology of learning (or, more accurately, behavior change) would agree with the generalization that the strength of a given behavior in any situation is a function of the similarity of the current situation to that existing when the behavior was learned. When environments vary considerably, the transfer of learning is usually minimal. Thus, for example, an animal trained to approach an object in an experimental apparatus will probably ignore the same object when it is presented elsewhere.

In our everyday life we show an implicit understanding of this process. If a child hurts his leg in learning to ride a bicycle, we do not try to teach him to ride better while he is still using crutches. Yet, our prison system defies both the scientific literature and our commonsense knowledge of the principles of behavioral change.

When a prisoner is released, he returns to the very different conditions presented by the free world, where he must structure his own life, choices are required, many aspects of the environment are highly variable, and the range of possible behaviors is much greater than in prison. Whatever is learned in prison is mostly no longer applicable, because of the difference between the environments. As a result, even if he did acquire different behaviors in prison, that learning would not easily transfer to the outside world. If men are sent to prison because of deficiencies in their behavioral control mechanisms on the outside, they are not likely to display the necessary control after they are released. Good intentions notwithstanding, to expect criminal offenders to change their behavior on the outside while confined to a cell is at best chimerical.

The specificity of behaviors to environments is a well-known phenomenon, and we experience it daily. We may notice that we behave slightly differently in each of the situations that comprise our lives. We act differently toward our children than we do toward our co-workers, differently to a spouse than to a supervisor. Many of us have experienced a return to parents' homes after an extended absence, and noticed how the feelings of strangeness change almost immediately into familiarity, and how one's behavioral role can return to that of a child despite one's age and normal role in other environments.

So, our behavior varies considerably across situations, and we are each capable of playing several very different roles. When we return to a familiar environment from which we have been absent for a while, the power of environmental contingencies, old stimuli working old habits, memory, and a variety of other factors, all act in concert to return our behavior very quickly to what it had been before in that environment. Although examples of this sort of switching are easily observable in everyday life, one must consider how much more powerful is the effect for a person making the transition from prison to the outside world. Virtually every aspect of the external environment changes, along with rules, regulations, procedures, and the conventions and expectations of ordinary social interaction. As well, there is a complete change of the people whom the prisoner sees, and an entirely different set of problems to cope with.

The difference between prison and the outside world thus defines a radical transition for the inmate released directly to the street. The result is a quick behavioral change of state, with a minimum of transfer from one environment to the other. Even if anything had been learned in prison, there would be little carryover after release. Even more, people who have made the transition several times could learn to make the switch immediately, with no transfer whatsoever.

This helps to explain why the prospect of change is lowest among men who have been imprisoned several times. Recidivists do not change as a result of prison, because in effect they lead two lives, compartmentalized and separate from each other. Although they do not like returning to prison, the criminal justice system has no way of interrupting their pattern of criminal behaviors except to return them to prison, but this cuts them off from their life on the outside and can provide no basis for changing the undesirable behaviors.

Changing the Prison Experience

We are led to argue that there need to be some major changes in what inmates experience in prison. First, there must be programs designed explicitly to teach coping skills, including both short-term ways of mitigating problems and long-term planning and organizational strategies. These programs should be available to all inmates, and perhaps required for many, with successful completion considered in release plans. It should be emphasized that these programs would differ from any sort of program that we know to be currently available, e.g., life-skills training. They would include training in ways of analyzing problem situations, and evaluating and projecting the likely consequences of their actions. There would be training in such techniques as cognitive restructuring, problem-solving, covert responding, the use of anticipation, etc.

In addition, some attention must be given to the conditions for promoting transfer of new skills to life on the outside after release. The problem of the conditions for transfer of learning has not previously been dealt with in the correctional literature, but a number of behavioral researchers have been concerned with it, both for theoretical reasons and for the purpose of maximizing therapeutic gains. Transfer can be increased by the use of particular strategies such as the use of gradual transitions from the original training situation to the target environment. Thus, we must stress the importance of graduated release programs, which allow inmates to alter some of their behaviors on the outside while still under the direct control and feedback of authorities. If such programs were made universal, and combined with programs aimed at teaching offenders better ways of coping with problems and of organizing and planning their lives, then we would expect that the extra investment would pay substantial dividends in improved effectiveness of the correctional system.

Until this happens, we do not see much chance for improvements in the effectiveness of the prison system at changing the behavior of inmates after release. We conclude that prisons do not do the damage some have claimed, but neither do they help at all. Rather, they act as very expensive ways to isolate miscreants from the rest of us, holding them in suspension, behaviorally frozen until they resume their lives for better or worse after release.

As a result, prisoners are released no better than when they entered. Whatever the good intentions of both staff and inmates, our data lead us to predict that the effects of prisons will inevitably be small and recidivism high. In this view, previous analyses have not dealt with the central problem. Until changes are made, we shall all continue to pay the price.

References

Abbott, J.H.
  1981 In the Belly of the Beast. New York: Random House.
Akers, R., N.S. Hayner, and W. Gruninger
  1977 "Prisonization in five countries: type of prison and inmate characteristics." Criminology 4: 527–554.
Alper, B.S.
  1974 Prison Inside-out. Cambridge, MA: Ballinger Publishing Co.
Alpert, G.P.
  1979 "Patterns of change in prisonization: a longitudinal analysis." Criminal Justice and Behavior 6: 159–174.
Anderson, C.R.
  1977 "Locus of control, coping behaviors, and performance in a stress setting: a longitudinal study." Journal of Applied Psychology 62: 446–451.
Andrews, D.A., and J.S. Wormith
  1983 Criminal Sentiments, Criminological Theory, and Criminal Behavior: A Construct Validation. Ottawa: Carleton University. Unpublished manuscript.
Atchley, R.C., and M.P. McCabe
  1968 "Socialization in correctional communities: a replication." American Sociological Review 33: 774–785.
Austin, J., and B. Krisberg
  1985 "Incarceration in the United States: the extent and future of the problem." Annals of the American Academy of Political and Social Science 478: 15–30.
Bandura, A.
  1978 "The self-system in reciprocal determinism." American Psychologist 33: 344–358.
Banister, P.A., F.V. Smith, K.J. Heskin, and N. Bolton
  1973 "Psychological correlates of long-term imprisonment: I. cognitive variables." British Journal of Criminology 3: 312–323.
Beck, A.T.
  1967 Depression: Clinical, Experimental and Theoretical Aspects. New York: Hoeber.
Beck, A.T.
  1976 Cognitive Theory and the Emotional Disorders. New York: International

Universities Press.

Beck, A.T., M. Kovacs, and A. Weissman
1979 "Assessment of suicidal intention: the scale for suicide ideation." Journal of Consulting and Clinical Psychology 47: 343–352.

Beck, A.T., A. Weismann, D. Lester, and L. Trexler
1974 "The measurement of pessimism: the Hopelessness Scale." Journal of Consulting and Clinical Psychology 42: 861–865.

Bennett, L.A.
1974 "The application of self-esteem measures in a correctional setting: II. changes in self-esteem during incarceration." Journal of Research in Crime and Delinquency 1: 9–15.

Berk, R.
1966 "Organizational goals and inmates' organization." American Journal of Sociology 71: 522–534.

Blumstein, A.
1986 "Sentencing and the prison crowding problem." In S.D. Gottfredson and S. McConville (eds.) America's Correctional Crisis: Prison Populations and Public Policy. New York: Greenwood Press.

Bolton, N., F.V. Smith, K.J. Heskin, and P.A. Banister
1976 "Psychological correlates of long-term imprisonment." British Journal of Criminology 16: 38–47.

Bonta, J.
1986 "Prison crowding: searching for the functional correlates." American Psychologist 41: 99–101.

Bonta, J., and P. Gendreau
1987 Re-examining the Cruel and Unusual Punishment of Prison Life. Unpublished manuscript.

Bowers, K.S.
1973 "Situationism in psychology: an analysis and critique." Psychological Review 80: 307–336.

Bowker, L.H.
1977 Prison Subcultures. Lexington, MA: Lexington Books.

Bukstel, L.H., and P.R. Kilmann
1980 "Psychological effects of imprisonment on confined individuals." Psychological Review 88: 469–493.

Bureau of Justice Statistics
1985 Prisoners in 1984. Washington, DC: U.S. Department of Justice.

Caron, R.
1978 Go Boy: Memories of a Life Behind Bars. Toronto: McGraw-Hill.

Chaiken, J.M., and M.R. Chaiken
1982 Varieties of Criminal Behavior: Summary and Policy Implications. Santa Monica, CA: Rand Corporation.

Clayton, T.
1970 Men in Prison. London: Hamish Hamilton.

Clemmer, D.
1950 "Observations on imprisonment as a source of criminality." Journal of Criminal Law, Criminology and Police Science 41: 311–319.
1958 The Prison Community. New York: Holt, Rinehart, and Winston. (Originally published 1940.)

Cline, H.
    1968   "The determinants of normative patterns in correctional institutions." In
           J. Christie (ed.) Scandinavian Studies in Criminology II. Oslo: Oslo Uni-
           versity Press.
Cohen, S., and L. Taylor
    1981   Psychological Survival: The Experience of Long-term Imprisonment,
           Second edition, Harmondsworth, England: Penguin.
Communications Division
    1984   Report of the Advisory Committee to the Solicitor General of Canada
           on the Management of Correctional Institutions. Ottawa: Solicitor
           General of Canada.
Coopersmith, S.
    1967   The Antecedents of Self-Esteem. San Francisco: W.H. Freeman.
Corrections Services in Canada, 1980–81
    1982   Ottawa: Statistics Canada.
Crowne, D.P., and D.A. Marlowe
    1960   "New scale of social desirability independent of psychopathology." Jour-
           nal of Consulting Psychology 24: 349–354.
Culbertson, R.G.
    1975   "The effects of institutionalization on the delinquent inmate's self-
           concept." Journal of Criminal Law and Criminology 66: 83–93.
Cullen, F.T.
    1983   Rethinking Crime and Deviance Theory: The Emergence of a Structuring
           Tradition. Totowa, NJ: Rowman and Allanheld.
Cullen, F.T., and K.E. Gilbert
    1982   Reaffirming Rehabilitation. Cincinnati, OH: Anderson.
Dohrenwend, B.S., and B.P. Dohrenwend
    1973   Stressful Life Events: Their Nature and Effects. New York: Wiley.
Driscoll, P.J.
    1952   "Factors related to the institutional adjustment of prison inmates." Jour-
           nal of Abnormal and Social Psychology 47: 593–596.
Ellis, D.
    1984   "Crowding and prison violence: integration of research and theory."
           Criminal Justice and Behavior 11: 277–308.
Ellis, A., and R. Grieger (eds.)
    1977   Handbook of Rational Emotive Therapy. New York: Springer.
Estes, W.K. (ed.)
    1975   Handbook of Learning and Cognitive Processes: Vol 1. Introduction to
           Concepts and Issues. New York: Halsted.
Faine, J.R.
    1973   "A self-consistency approach to prisonization." Sociological Quarterly 4:
           576–588.
Farrington, D.P.
    1979   "Longitudinal research on crime and delinquency." In N. Morris and M.
           Tonry (eds.), Crime and Justice vol. 1. Chicago: University of Chicago
           Press.
Farrington, D.P., L.E. Ohlin, and J.Q. Wilson
    1986   Understanding and Controlling Crime: Toward a New Research Strategy.
           New York: Springer.

Fichtler, H., R.R. Zimmerman, and R.T. Moore
  1973 "Comparison of self-esteem of prison and nonprison groups." Perceptual and Motor Skills 36: 39–44.
Flanagan, T.J.
  1980 "The pains of long-term imprisonment." British Journal of Criminology 20: 148–156.
  1982 "Lifers and long-termers: doing big time." In R. Johnson and H. Toch (eds.), The Pains of Imprisonment. Beverly Hills, CA: Sage.
Gaes, G.G.
  1985 "The effects of overcrowding in prison." In M. Tonry and N. Morris (eds.), Crime and Justice, vol. 6. Chicago: University of Chicago Press.
Garabedian, P.C.
  1963 "Social roles and processes of socialization in the prison community." Social Problems 11: 139–152.
  1964 "Social roles in a correctional community." Journal of Criminal Law, Criminology, and Police Science 55: 235–247.
Garry, E.
  1984 Options to Justice Crowding. Washington, DC: U.S. National Institute of Justice.
Gearing, M.L.
  1979 "The MMPI as a primary differentiator and predictor of behavior in prison: a methodological critique and review of the recent literature." Psychological Bulletin 86: 929–963.
Gendreau, P., and J. Bonta
  1984 "Solitary confinement is not cruel and unusual punishment: people sometimes are!" Canadian Journal of Criminology 26: 467–478.
Gendreau, P., and M. Gibson
  1970 "The development of attitudinal, behavioral, and social-historical measures for prediction, classification and treatment." Project 22. Toronto: Ontario Ministry of Correctional Services.
Gendreau, P., M. Gibson, C.T. Surridge, and J.J. Hug
  1973 "Self-esteem changes associated with six months' imprisonment." Proceedings of the Canadian Congress of Criminology and Corrections, 81–89.
Gendreau, P., B.A. Grant, and M. Leipciger
  1979 "Self-esteem, incarceration, and recidivism." Criminal Justice and Behavior 6: 67–75.
Gibbs, J.J. Maiello, L.A. Kolb, K.S., Garofolo, J., Adler, F., and Costello, S.R.
  1985 Stress, Setting and Satisfaction: The Final Report of the Man-Jail Transactions Project. Washington, DC: National Institute of Justice. NCJR 95317.
Glaser, D.
  1964 The Effectiveness of a Prison and Parole System. Indianapolis, IN: Bobbs-Merrill.
Goffman, E.
  1961 Asylums: Essays on the Social Situation of Mental Patients and Other Inmates. Garden City, NJ: Anchor.
Goodstein, L.
  1979 "Inmate adjustment to prison and transition to community life." Journal

of Research in Crime and Delinquency 16: 246–272.

Gottfredson, S.D.
1986   "The dynamics of prison populations." Paper prepared for the working group on Jail and Prison Crowding, Committee on Research in Law Enforcement and the Administration of Justice, (U.S.) National Academy of Sciences.

Gottfredson, S.D., and S. McConville (eds.)
1986   America's Correctional Crisis: Prison Populations and Public Policy. New York: Greenwood Press.

Gunderson, E.K.E., and R.H. Rahe (eds.)
1974   Life Events and Illness. Springfield, IL: Charles C. Thomas.

Haley, K.R.
1983   Problems and Coping Behavior in Fourth-year University Undergraduates. Unpublished B.A. (Honors) thesis, Queen's University at Kingston.

Hawkins, G.
1976   The Prison: Policy and Practice. Chicago: University of Chicago Press.

Heather, N.
1977   "Personal illness in 'lifers' and the effects of long-term indeterminate sentences." British Journal of Criminology 17: 378–386.

Heffernan, E.
1972   Making It in Prison: The Square, the Cool, and the Life. New York: Wiley.

Helson, H.
1964   Adaptation-Level Theory: An Experimental and Systematic Approach to Behavior. New York: Harper and Row.

Hepburn, J.R., and J.R. Stratton
1977   "Total institutions and inmate self-esteem." British Journal of Criminology 7: 237–250.

Heskin, K.J., N. Bolton, F.V. Smith, and P.A. Banister
1974   "Psychological correlates of long-term imprisonment III: attitudinal variables." British Journal of Criminology 14: 150–157.

Heskin, K.J., F.V. Smith, P.A. Banister and N. Bolton
1973   "Psychological correlates of long-term imprisonment: II. personality variables." British Journal of Criminology 13: 323–330.

Hoffman, P.B.
1983   "Screening for risk: a revised salient factor score (SFS81)." Journal of Criminal Justice 11: 539–547.

Inform
1985   Ottawa: Offender Information Systems, Corrections Service of Canada.

Irwin, J.
1970   The Felon. Englewood Cliffs, NJ: Prentice Hall.
1980   Prisons in Turmoil. Toronto: Little Brown and Co.

Irwin, J., and D. Cressey
1962   "Thieves, convicts, and the inmate subculture." Social Problems 10: 142–155.

Jackson, D.N.
1976   The Basic Personality Inventory. London, Ontario: Research Psychologists Press.

Jackson, M.
  1983 Prisoners of Isolation: Solitary Confinement in Canada. Toronto: University of Toronto Press.

Jacobs, J.
  1976 "Stratification and conflict among prison inmates." Journal of Criminal Law and Criminology 66: 476–482.

Jaman, D.
  1971 Behavior During the First year in Prison. Research report No. 32. Sacramento, CA: California Department of Corrections.

Jensen, G.F., and D. Jones
  1976 "Perspectives in immate culture: a study of women in prison." Social Forces 54: 590–603.

Johnson, R.
  1976 Culture and Crisis in Confinement. Lexington MA: Lexington Books.
  1987 Hard Time: Understanding and Reforming the Prison. Monterey, CA: Brooks/Cole.

Johnson, R., and H. Toch
  1982 The Pains of Imprisonment. Beverly Hills, CA: Sage.

Kanner, A.D., J.C. Coyne, C. Schaefer, and R.S. Lazarus
  1981 "Comparison of two modes of stress measurement: daily hassles and uplifts versus major life events." Journal of Behavioral Medicine 4: 1–39.

Kassebaum, G., D. Ward and D. Wilner
  1971 Prison Treatment and Parole Survival. New York: Wiley.

Lazarus, R.S.
  1966 Psychological Stress and the Coping Process. New York: McGraw Hill.
  1980 "The stress and coping paradigm." In C. Eisdorfer, D. Cohen, A. Kleinman, and P. Maxim (eds.), Theoretical Bases for Psychopathology. New York: Spectrum.

Lazarus, R.S., J.R. Averill, and E.M. Opton
  1970 "Toward a cognitive theory of emotion." In M.B. Arnold (ed.), Feelings and Emotions. New York: Academic Press.

Lazarus, R.S., and S. Folkman
  1983 Stress, Appraisal, and Coping. New York: Springer.

Lazarus, R.S., and R. Launier
  1978 "Stress-related transactions between person and environment." In L.A. Pervin and M. Lewis (eds.), Internal and External Determinants of Behavior. New York: Plenum.

Lightfoot-Barbaree, L., and H. Barbaree
  1979 Drug Use Inventory. Queen's University at Kingston. Unpublished manuscript.

Lipsky, M.
  1980 Street Level Bureaucracy: Dilemmas of the Individual in Public Services. New York: Russell Sage Foundation.

Little, V.L., and P.C. Kendall
  1979 "Cognitive-behavioral interventions with delinquents: problem solving, role-taking, and self-control." In P.C. Kendall and S.D. Hollon (eds.), Cognitive-Behavioral Interventions: Theory, Research and Procedures. New York: Academic Press.

MacKenzie, D.L., and L. Goodstein
 1985 "Long-term incarceration impacts and characteristics of long-term offend-
        ers: an empirical analysis." Criminal Justice and Behavior 12: 395–414.
Magnussen, D., and N.S. Endler (eds.)
 1977 Personality at the Crossroads: Current Issues in Interactional Psychology.
        Hillsdale, NJ: Lawrence Erlbaum Associates.
Manocchio, A.J., and J. Dunn
 1970 The Time Game: Two Views of Prison. Beverly Hills, CA: Sage.
McKay, H.B., C.H.S. Jayewardene, and P.B. Reedie
 1977 Report on the Effects of Long-term Incarceration and a Proposed
        Strategy for Future Research. Contract report for Ministry of the Solicitor
        General of Canada.
McNair, D.M., M. Lorr, and L.F. Droppleman
 1971 Manual: Profile of Mood States. San Diego, CA.: Educational and In-
        dustrial Testing Service.
Meichenbaum, D.
 1977 Cognitive-Behavior Modification: An Integrative Approach. New York:
        Plenum Press.
Miller, S., and S. Dinitz
 1973 "Measuring institutional impact, a follow-up." Criminology 11: 417–426.
Mischel, W.
 1973 "Toward a cognitive social-learning reconceptualization of personality."
        Psychological Review 80: 252–283.
Moos, R. (ed.)
 1976 Human Adaptation: Coping with Life Crises. Lexington, MA: Heath.
Morris, T., and P. Morris
 1963 Pentonville: A Sociological Study of an English Prison. London: Rout-
        ledge and Kagan Paul.
Myers, T.
 1982 "Alcohol and violent crime re-examined: self-reports from two sub-
        groups of Scottish male prisoners." British Journal of Addiction 77: 399–
        413.
Nuffield, J.
 1982 Parole Decision-Making in Canada: Research Towards Decision Guide-
        lines. Ottawa: Ministry of the Solicitor General of Canada.
Offord, D.R.
 1982 "Family backgrounds of male and female delinquents." In J. Gunn and
        D.P. Farrington (eds.), Abnormal Offenders, Delinquency, and the
        Criminal Justice System. Chichester, England: Wiley.
Pell, E. (ed.)
 1972 Maximum Security: Letters from Prison. New York: E.P. Dutton.
Poole, E.D., and R.M. Regoli
 1983 "Violence in juvenile institutions." Criminology 21; 213–232.
Poole, E.D., R.M. Regoli, and C.W. Thomas
 1980 "The measurement of inmate social role types: an assessment" Journal of
        Criminal Law and Criminology 71: 317–324.
Porporino, F.J.
 1983 Coping Behavior in Prison Inmates: Description and Correlates. Unpub-
        lished Ph.D. thesis, Queen's University at Kingston.

Rasch, W.
  1977 "The development of the mental and physical state of persons sentenced to life imprisonment." In S. Rizkalla, R. Levy, and R. Zauberman (eds.), Long-term Imprisonment: An International Seminar. Centre International de Criminologie Comparée, Université de Montreal.
  1981 "The effects of indeterminate sentencing: a study of men sentenced to life imprisonment." International Journal of Law and Psychiatry 4: 417–431.
Reckless, W.C., and S. Dinitz
  1970 "Pioneering with self-concept as a vulnerability factor in delinquency." In Harwin Voss (ed.), Sociology, Delinquency and Delinquent Behavior. Boston: Little Brown.
Richards, B.
  1978 "The experience of long-term imprisonment." British Journal of Criminology 18: 162–169.
Rippere, V.
  1979 "Scaling the usefulness of antidepressive activities." Behavior Research and Therapy 17: 439–449.
Ross, R.R., and E.A. Fabiano
  1985 Time to Think: A Cognitive Model of Delinquency Prevention and Offender Rehabilitation. Johnson City, Tenn.: Institute of Social and Arts, Inc.
Rotter, J.
  1966 "Generalized expectancies of internal versus external control of reinforcement." Psychological Monographs 80, No. 609.
Sapsford, R.J.
  1978 "Life-sentence prisoners: psychological changes during sentence." British Journal of Criminology 18: 128–145.
  1983 Life Sentence Prisoners: Reaction, Response and change. Milton Keynes, England: Open University Press.
Sarason, I.G., J. Johnson, and J. Seigel
  1978 "Assessing the impact of life changes: development of the life experiences survey." Journal of Consulting and Clinical Psychology 46: 932–947.
Schrag, C.
  1954 "Leadership among prison inmates." American Sociological Review 19: 37–42.
  1961 "Some foundations for a theory of corrections." In D. Cressey (ed.), The Prison: Studies in Institutional Organization and Change. New York: Holt, Rinehart, and Winston.
Schwartz, B.
  1971 "Pre-institutional vs. situational influence in a correctional community." Journal of Criminal Law, Criminology, and Police Science 62: 530–545.
Shorer, C.E.
  1965 "The 'Ganser' syndrome." British Journal of Criminology 5: 120–131.
Smith, R.C., and C.D. Lay
  1974 "State and trait anxiety: an annotated bibliography." Psychological Reports 34: 519–594.
Spielberger, C.D., R.L. Gorsuch, and R.E. Lushene
  1970 Manual for the State-Trait Anxiety Inventory ("Self-Evaluation Questionnaire"). Palo Alto, CA: Consulting Psychologists Press.

Stokols, D.
   1972   "On the distinction between density and crowding." Psychological Re-
          view 79: 275–279.
Strahan, R., and K.C. Gerbasi
   1972   "Short, homogeneous version of the Marlowe-Crowne Social Desirability
          Scale." Journal of Clinical Psychology 28: 191–193.
Street, D.A.
   1965   "The inmate group in custodial and treatment settings." American
          Sociological Review 30: 40–55.
Suedfeld, P., C. Ramirez, J. Deaton, and G. Baker-Brown
   1982   "Reactions and attributes of prisoners in solitary confinement." Criminal
          Justice and Behavior 9: 303–340.
Sundstrom, E.
   1978   "Crowding as a sequential process: review of research on the effects
          of population density on humans." In A. Baum and M. Epstein (eds.),
          Human Response to Crowding. Hillsdale, NJ: Lawrence Erlbaum
          Associates.
Sykes, G.
   1958   The Society of Captives. Princeton, NJ: Princeton University Press.
Sykes, G.M., and S.L. Messinger,
   1960   "The inmate social system." In R. Cloward et al. (eds.), Theoretical
          Studies in Social Organization of the Prison. New York: Social Science
          Research Council.
Thomas, C.W.
   1977   "Theoretical perspectives on prisonization: a comparison of the importa-
          tion and deprivation models." Journal of Criminal law and Criminology
          68: 135–145.
   1987   Corrections in America: Problems of the Past and the Present. Beverly
          Hills, CA: Sage.
Thomas, C.W., and D.M. Petersen
   1977   Prison Organization and Inmate Subcultures. Indianapolis, IN: Bobbs-
          Merrill.
Thomas, C.W., D.M. Petersen, and R.M. Zingraff
   1978   "Structural and social psychological correlates of prisonization." Crimi-
          nology 16: 383–393.
Thomas, C.W., and E.D. Poole
   1975   "The consequences of incompatible goal structures in correctional set-
          tings." International Journal of Criminology and Penology 3: 27–42.
Thomas, C.W., and M.T. Zingraff
   1976   "Organizational structure as a determinant of prisonization." Pacific
          Sociological Review 19: 98–116.
Tittle, C.R.
   1972   "Institutional living and self-esteem." Social Problems 20: 65–77.
Tittle, C.R., and D.P. Tittle
   1964   "Social organization of prisoners: an empirical test." Social Forces 43:
          216–221.
Toch. H.
   1969   Violent Men: An Inquiry into the Psychology of Violence. Chicago:
          Aldine.

1975   Men in Crisis: Human Breakdowns in Prison. Chicago: Aldine.

1977   Living in Prison: The Ecology of Survival. New York: Macmillan.

Troyer, J.C., and D.E. Frease

1975   "Attitude change in a western Canadian penitentiary." Canadian Journal of Criminology and Corrections 7: 250–262.

Walker, N.

1983   "Side-effects of incarceration." British Journal of Criminology 23: 61–71.

Wellford, C.

1967   "Factors associated with adoption of the inmate code: a study of normative socialization." Journal of Criminal Law, Criminology, and Police Science 58: 197–203.

West, D.J., and D.P. Farrington

1973   Who Becomes Delinquent. London: Heinemann.

Wheeler, S.

1961   "Socialization in correctional communities." American Sociological Review 26: 696–712.

Wormith, J.S.

1980   "Training correctional volunteers for group discussions." Criminal Justice and Behavior 7: 341–356.

1984a "The controversy over the effects of long-term imprisonment." Canadian Journal of Criminology 26: 423–437.

1984b "Attitude and behavior change of correctional clientele: a three-year follow-up." Criminology 22: 595–618.

Zamble, E., F. Porporino, and J. Kalotay

1984   An Analysis of Coping Behavior in Prison Inmates. Programs Branch User Report No. 1984–77. Ottawa: Ministry of the Solicitor General of Canada.

Zamble, E., and F. Porporino

1980   An Analysis of Coping in Prison Inmates: Stage I Report. Contract report No. 62–6/5–206. Ottawa: Ministry of the Solicitor General of Canada.

Zingraff, M.T.

1980   "Inmate assimilation: a comparison of male and female delinquents." Criminal Justice and Behavior 7: 275–292.

Zuckerman, M., and B. Lubin

1965   Manual for the Multiple Affect Adjective Check List. San Diego, CA: Educational and Industrial Testing Serivces.

Appendices

TABLE A1. Significant correlations[a] of Social Desirability[b] scores with Self-Report measures.

Variable	Correlation
Interview measures	
Proportion of time dealing with outside	.21**
Proportion of time in group meetings	.19*
Proportion of time in passive activities	−.25**
Number of visits reported	.19*
Have general plan for doing time	−.17*
Frequency think of past	−.16*
Have sleep problem	−.15*
Questionnaire measures	
Drug frequency index	−.20*
Total number of drugs used	−.31***
Self-depreciation	−.69***
Self-esteem	.31***
Hopelessness	−.27**
Beck depression inventory	−.17*
Locus on control—external chance	−.18*

[a]This table includes significant correlations only. Values were computed for all other self-report measures used, but are not significant; quantitatively, this means that the correlation for any variable not included above is less than .15.
[b]Results reported here are for the Social Desirability scale at the first interview. Results for the second administration of the scale are similar, with about the same number of significant correlations overall, although only four of the measures listed above also had significant correlations with the Social Desirability scale at the second interview.
*$p < .05$
**$p < .01$
***$p < .001$

TABLE A2. Test-retest correlations for selected variables.

Variable	I1 vs I2	I1 vs I3
Coping Efficacy	.45***	.23***
Beck Depression Inventory	.25**	.13
Spielberger Trait Anxiety	.66***	.45***
Hopelessness Scale	.36***	.33***
Self-Esteem Scale	—	.18*
Locus of Control Scale (External)	—	.60***
Average sleeping time	.44***	.35***
Proportion of time in work	.23**	.11
Proportion of time in socializing	.22**	.38***
Proportion of time in visits and letters	.62***	.45***
Percent optional time in cell	.20*	.14
Number of friends	.40***	.42***
Number of letters	.38***	.31***
Frequency receive news	.53***	.46***
Frequency miss people from outside	.36***	.27***
Rating of current life	.30***	.27***

*$p < .05$
**$p < .01$
***$p < .001$

Coping Behavior Project

INFORMATION FORM

This sheet is intended to tell you about a study of inmate behavior in which we would like your cooperation. The study is aimed at finding out how people in prisons cope with their environment. It is being done by employees of the Department of Psychology at Queen's University, under the direction of Dr. Edward Zamble. It is being paid for by a contract with the Research Division of the Department of the Solicitor General.

In this study we will interview inmates as soon as possible after they come to the institution to which they are assigned. We will select the inmates to interview randomly, that is, according to chance. However, long-term inmates have a greater chance of being selected, since we especially want to find out about the effects of long-term imprisonment. The inmates selected will be asked about their behavior and experiences in and out of prison, and we will also ask them to fill out some questionnaires about the same things. We would also like to use some data which is available in their inmate files. Later, we will interview them again, to see what changes occur over time.

The purpose of the study is to get information on how prisons affect people. This could be used later in deciding how to improve the system. So, if you agree to cooperate, you will be helping us, and maybe also helping your fellow inmates. At the same time, we must tell you that we are only collecting information, so if you have any problems now, we cannot change anything for you, nor can we offer therapy. For those things, you will have to go through normal channels.

The results of the study will be included in a report to the sponsoring agency. All or part of the results will also be published separately in scientific journals, where they will be freely available for anyone to read. However, if you agree to participate, we will try to provide you with a copy of the summary of the results when we are finished. It would help if you would give us an address where you want it sent (in three years time).

All answers that inmates give will be strictly confidential, and they will be coded for all reports in such a way that no individual's answers can be identified. This confidentiality is guaranteed by the Canadian Human Rights Act, and we will also give our personal guarantees that it is respected. Also, the data will be used only for research purposes; if anyone ever wants to use them for any other purpose, we will require your written permission before we release any information.

CONSENT FORM

I, _____ (Name) have been asked to take part in a study of inmate behavior. I have been given an "Information Form" describing the study, which is being done in the Department of Psychology at Queen's University under the direction of Dr. Edward Zamble.

I agree to take part in this study, and to be interviewed about my experiences in and out of prison. I will try to answer questions to the best of my memory, but I understand that my taking part in this study is purely voluntary, and that I am free to refuse to answer specific questions; I may also withdraw from the study if I feel it necessary. My participation in this study will not count for or against me in any way.

After the interview I will be asked to fill out some questionnaires about my behavior and experiences, and I also agree to do this. I will also be asked for a further interview in about three months time, and again a year later, to see how I am getting along at those times. I also agree to allow these researchers to obtain additional information from my institutional and medical files.

Any information I give will be strictly confidential. Nothing I say will affect my position here in any way. The information I give will be used for scientific purposes, in order to better understand how imprisonment affects people. My answers will be coded in such a way that I cannot be identified in any report of the results.

My signature below indicates that I have read the above, and that I agree to take part and give my consent to the researchers having access to my institutional and medical files. The interviewer will also sign to guarantee the conditions stated above.

_____

date   inmate's signature

_____

date   interviewer's signature

To help us send your copy of our summary report, please give an address below where it is likely you can be reached in three years.

_____
_____
_____

Coping Interview I

PROCEDURE

(The inmate will be called up. The purpose of the study will be explained, and he will be given the consent forms to read and sign. If he agrees to participate, the interview will proceed. The inmate will be offered coffee and cigarettes.)

INTRODUCTION

Let me explain to you the areas that I want to ask you about. First, we want to get some background information. Then, we want to know about your life on the outside: we want to know how you lived, the problems you faced, and, especially, how you dealt with problems. Finally, we want to know the same sorts of things about your life in prison, that is, problems and how you deal with them.

PART A. BACKGROUND INFORMATION

First, let me get some background information. I could get some of this from your file, but it's probably easier to get it right from you.

001.   How old are you?

002.   a. How long is your sentence? (__ years, __months)
       b. For what? _____ (offense)
       c. How much time have you already been in prison since you were
           arrested on this charge? (__ months)
       d. Before your trial, how much time did you EXPECT you would
           get? (__ months)

003.   Do you have any APPEALS coming up? (Yes, No)
       IF YES
       a. Are you appealing the CONVICTION or the SENTENCE?
       IF CONVICTION
       b. What are the chances of the appeal being successful? (__ %)
       c. How often do you THINK about the appeal? (all the time, most of
           the time, sometimes, rarely, never)
       IF SENTENCE
       d. What are the chances of the appeal being successful? (__ %)
       e. If it is successful, how long do you expect the reduced sentence
           will be? (__ years, __ months)
       f. How often do you THINK about the appeal? (all the time, most of
           the time, sometimes, rarely, never)

004. If you present sentence remains UNCHANGED, how much time do you actually EXPECT TO SERVE? (___ months)
    a. Is that a LONG time? (Yes, No)

005. What do you think are the CHANCES you may be released after 1/3 of your sentence, that is, at the EARLIEST possible time? (___ %) (N.B. FOR LIFE TERM, OMIT REFERENCE TO 1/3 SENTENCE.)
    b. What do you think are the CHANCES you might not be released until you have served 2/3 of your sentence, that is, the MANDA-TORY release date? (___ %) (N.B. FOR LIFE TERM, CHANGE TO "YOU MIGHT NEVER BE RELEASED".)

006. Were you ever in a penitentiary BEFORE? (Yes, No)
    IF YES,
    a. HOW OLD were you when you first went in?
    (___ Years)
    b. HOW MANY terms did you serve? (___ terms)
    c. HOW LONG were you there each time? (list terms, months each ___, ___, ___, ___)
    d. Were you ever in a REFORMATORY or training school? (Yes, No)
    IF YES
    e. How OLD were you when you first went in?
    (___/years)
    f. How many TERMS did you serve? (___#)
    g. How LONG were you there each time? (list terms, months each ___, ___, ___, ___)

007. Have you ever been in any OTHER INSTITUTIONS, for example hospital? (Minimum of one month) (Yes, No)
    IF YES,
    a. What KIND of institution? (_____ Type)
    b. HOW LONG were you there? (___ terms; ___ total months)

008. Have you ever been treated for PSYCHIATRIC or emotional prob-lems? (Yes, No)
    IF YES,
    a. BY WHOM? (Type of professional _____)
    b. For WHAT? (Diagnosis or symptoms _____)
    c. For HOW LONG? (___ months)

009. Have you ever seriously thought of SUICIDE? (Yes, No)
    IF YES,
    a. HOW OFTEN? (___ times in last year)
    b. How you ever considered HOW you would do it if you did try? (Yes, No)

IF YES,
c. Have you ever actually ATTEMPTED suicide? (Yes, No)
IF YES,
d. How MANY times? (__#)

010. Have you ever had any serious physical or HEALTH problems?
(Yes, No)
IF YES,
a. WHAT? (Type _____)
b. It is still CURRENT? (Yes, No)
IF YES,
c. HOW LONG have you had this (these) problem(s)?

d. Is it being TREATED? (Yes, No)

011. Are you on any MEDICATION now? (Yes, No)
IF YES,
a. WHAT? (Name or type _____)
b. For what REASON? (Type _____)

012. How far did you go in SCHOOL? (Grade __)
IF LESS THAN GRADE 11,
a. HOW OLD were you when you quit? (__ years)

013. Do you have a FAMILY outside? (Yes, No)
IF YES,
a. WHO are the people in it? (List)

014. Are your PARENTS living? (Yes, no)
IF NO,
a. WHICH of them is alive? (Mother, Father, Neither)
b. How OLD were you when (deceased parent) died?
(__ years)
c. What is (was) your father's occupation? (Specify)
IF EITHER ARE ALIVE,
d. When did you LAST LIVE WITH your parents?
(__ years old)

015. Do you have any BROTHERS or SISTERS? (Yes, No)
IF YES,
a. How many BROTHERS? (__)
b. How many SISTERS? (__)
c. List birth order.
d. Have any of them ever been in PRISON? (Yes, No)
IF YES,
e. HOW MANY? (# __)

PART B. OUTSIDE PRISON

Now I would like a picture of your life outside in the 6 months before you were arrested for your current offense. (If inmate was in prison during this time, use most recent period of one continuous month outside.)
IN THE 6 MONTHS BEFORE YOU WERE ARRESTED:

001. Were you living ALONE or were you living with other people?
 IF WITH OTHER PEOPLE,
 a. WHO? (__ # of persons; M or F; relationships)
 b. HOW Long had you been living with that (those) person(s)? (__ months)
 IF LIVING WITH A WOMAN,
 c. Were you MARRIED to her? (Yes, No; N.B. Common-law married)
 d. For how long?
 e. Were you ever married to ANYONE ELSE (Yes, No)
 IF YES,
 f. When did you LAST LIVE WITH your previous wife? (Date __)
 IF NOT LIVING WITH WOMAN,
 g. Were you EVER married? (Yes, no)
 h. Did you have any steady RELATIONSHIPS with women in the period just before your arrest?
 IF YES,
 i. HOW MANY? (# __)
 j. HOW LONG had you been going with her (them)? (__ months)
 IF NO,
 k. Did you EVER have a steady relationship with a woman?
 IF YES
 l. When did the LAST relationship end? (__ months-ago)
 IF NO
 m. WHY NOT? (Reason _____)

002. Do you have any CHILDREN? (Yes, No)
 IF YES,
 a. HOW MANY? (# __)
 b. Did they all LIVE WITH you? (Yes, No)
 IF NO,
 c. HOW MANY lived with you? (# __)

003. Did you LIVE IN a house or an apartment? How big was it? (__ number of bedrooms)

004. Did you have any close FRIENDS? (Yes, No)
 IF YES,
 a. HOW MANY? (# __)

b. How many of those close friends were involved in CRIMINAL ACTIVITIES? (# __)

c. What about other people you knew who weren't close friends: what percentage of them were involved in criminal activities? (__ %)

Now I'd like to talk about how you occupied your time. IN THE 6 MONTHS BEFORE YOUR ARREST OR MOST RECENT PERIOD OUTSIDE:

005. How much time did you SLEEP usually? (__ hours)

a. Did you have any PROBLEMS SLEEPING? (Yes, No)

IF YES,

b. WHAT? (Elucidate symptoms and reasons if possible; distinguish especially getting to sleep from early waking.)

c. Did you use any DRUGS to help you sleep? (Yes, No)

d. Did you ever sleep during the DAY? (Yes, No)

IF YES,

e. Would you describe this as NAPPING or longer sleep periods? (napping, longer (average hours __/day)

006. In terms of work, were you TRAINED to do any special kind of job? (Yes, No)

IF YES,

a. WHAT sort of work? (Specify _____)

007. Were you WORKING? (Yes, No)

IF YES,

a. What KIND of job was it? (Specify)

b. HOW LONG had been doing that job? (__ months)

c. How did you FEEL about the job? Rate on a 100-point scale, where 0 is "couldn't stand it" and 100 is "the best job that could be" (Rating: ____)

IF NOT WORKING,

d. How did you SUPPORT yourself? (Specify)

e. When did you LAST work? (elapsed time __ months)

f. What was your LONGEST PERIOD of employment? (__ months)

g. Doing WHAT? (Specify)

I'd like to get a general picture of how you divided your TIME. I have a number of categories here, and I'd like to find out how much time you spent on each. First, I'll read you the whole list, and then I will go over them one at a time.

008. Aside from sleeping, how much of your TIME did you spend on each of the following (we would like the number of hours in an average week)

a. WORK or school (__ hours/week)
b. FAMILY, that is, people listed before.
    (__ hours/week)
c. With FRIENDS, or socializing (__ hours/week)
d. TV, listening to radio or music (__ hours/week)
e. SPORTS and hobbies (__ hours/week)
f. OTHER things (may include criminal activities) (__ hours/week)
(If more than 3 hours/week in categories e. or f., then specify. It is
possible that the total of hours is more than that available in a week;
this is permissible but it should be checked with the respondent first.)

009. What were your FAVORITE activities on the outside? (Specify, rate
     enjoyment on 100-point scale, where 0 is "couldn't care less" and 100
     is "the best that could be").
     Item. . . . . Rating. . . . .
     1.
     2.
     3.
     4.
     5.
     IF LESS THAN 3 ITEMS, RESTATE:
     (Insert answers in above table; indicate from restated question.)
     a. What were the things that gave you the MOST PLEASURE, that
         you most liked to do? (Specify; rate on same scale)

010. Did you KEEP IN TOUCH with current events while you were out-
     side? (Yes, No)
     a. How often did you LISTEN TO NEWS on the radio or TV? (__/
         week)
     b. How often did you READ newspapers or news-magazines? (__/
         week)

Now I'd like to see what PROBLEMS you had on the outside and what
you did when they happened.

011. Were there any PROBLEMS that stand out from what you remem-
     ber about your life on the outside? (Specify)
     IF YES,
     (Those problems mentioned above may be omitted from list below.)
Well, there are many common problems that occur for guys on the outside.
I'd like to ask you about some of those; we have problems organized in a
couple of general areas, AND I'D LIKE TO GO OVER THEM ONE AT
A TIME; WOULD YOU ANSWER IN TERMS OF THE PERIOD
WE'VE BEEN TALKING ABOUT, THAT IS, THE 6 MONTHS BE-
FORE YOUR ARREST.

I. The External Environment

The first area includes general situations and things in your environment. Let's start by talking about work.

012. What sort of PROBLEMS did you have at WORK (when you were working)? (Specify.)
(Problems regarding people should be deferred to questions below (18–20). If the interviewee responds with problems of this sort here, say "We'll talk about that shortly; right now I want to know about general problems in the work situation.")
IF NO JOB AT THAT TIME,
a. Was NOT HAVING A JOB a problem for you? (Yes, No)
IF YES,
b. WHY? (Specify)

013. Was MONEY a problem? (Yes, No)
IF YES,
a. How?

014. How about specific things in your living arrangements? Did you feel CROWDED or that you had too little PRIVACY? (Yes, No)

015. Did you feel that things were too NOISY or that you couldn't get peace and quiet? (Yes, No)

016. Were there any OTHER problems in your environment that affected you? (Yes, No)
IF YES,
a. WHAT? (Specify)

II. Interpersonal

The next general area covers problems with PEOPLE.
IF HE HAD A JOB,
017. Let's start with work. What problems did you have with your BOSS or supervisors? (Specify)

018. What about OTHER PEOPLE you worked with: how did you get along with them? (specify problems)

019. Was there any OTHER person or situation at work that created problems for you? (Yes, No)
IF YES,
a. WHAT was the problem? (Specify)

IF HE LIVED WITH A WOMAN (OR MARRIED) ASK:
020. How about people at HOME? What problems did you have with your WIFE (or woman friend)? (Specify)

IF HE LIVED WITH CHILDREN, ASK:

021. What problems did you have with the KIDS? (Specify)

IF HE LIVED WITH OTHERS, ASK:

022. How did you get along with __? (Specify)

023. Was there anyone ELSE you had a problem with, for example a neighbor or someone else? (Yes, No)
    IF YES,
    a. WHAT was the problem? (Specify)

024. Did you have any problems with your FRIENDS? (Specify)
    a. Did you have ENOUGH friends? (Yes, No)
    b. Was LONELINESS a problem? (Yes, No)
    c. Did you have someone you were CLOSE TO to talk with? (Yes, No)
    IF YES,
    d. WHO? (Specify)

III. Internal

The last area people have problems with is their thoughts. Sometimes these are very specific and sometimes they are very general. For example you might get upset because you think you didn't go far enough in school in math—that would be specific; or you might think your life was unbearable—that would be general.

025. In the period we've been talking about, what THOUGHTS did you have about life and about yourself? (Specify)

IF NECESSARY, GIVE EXAMPLES:
    a. Well, you MIGHT HAVE THOUGHT that things were going your way, or that you were really in control of your life; on the other hand, you might have thought that you were a victim of more than your share of bad luck, or that you yourself were a loser. Did you ever think of any of these or similar things?
    IF YES,
    b. WHAT? (Specify)

IF NO CLEAR ANSWER, RESTATE:
    c. Suppose somebody had asked you to DESCRIBE YOURSELF in one or two words at that time. How would you have done it? (Answer should be confined to general evaluative and efficacy considerations, not physical or socioeconomic description.)

0.26. Now, we have a number of different problems. Of these, some might have been important to you at the time, and others may not have mattered very much at all. Can you tell me which were the MOST IMPORTANT? First, I'll read off all the problems I have noted.

Then, I'd like you to rank them for me, picking the most important
first and so on. (Up to $n = 5$)

Rank. . . . . .Item. . . . .

1.

2.

3.

4.

5

IF HE CAN'T RANK, USE PAIRWISE COMPARISONS TO CON-
STRUCT ORDER

027. When you had a problem, who were you likely to turn to for HELP?
      (Self, spouse, family, friend, professional (Specify))

IF "IT DEPENDS" (give highest ranked problem as example).

Coping Analysis

(From the problems listed above, three should be chosen if possible; an
absolute minimum of two is required. Problems chosen should be in different areas, for which it is likely that different emotional responses are involved. Choose the highest ranked problems meeting these requirements.
The questions below are repeated three times, once for each problem. They
should be considered as an outline for inquiry rather than rigidly specified,
since many of them are not appropriate for some problems, and some of the
information requested may not be accessible to the respondent.)

Now I'd like to find out what you did when these problems occurred. Let's
consider them one at a time.

028. When __ (first problem) occurred, how did it make you FEEL?
      (Specify)
      IF NO CLEAR ANSWER,
      a.   Did you feel ANGRY? (Yes, No)
      b.   Did you feel DEPRESSED or low? (Yes, No)
      c.   Did you feel ANXIOUS or uptight? (Yes, No)
      d.   Did you feel GUILTY or ashamed? (Yes, No)
      IF MORE THAN ONE,
      e.   Which did you feel MORE of? (Specify)

029. (DIRECT ACTION) When this happened, and you felt that way,
      WHAT DID YOU DO right then? (Specify)
      a.   What happened THEN? (Specify)

      OMIT PARTS OF THE FOLLOWING SEQUENCES WHICH
      ARE ANSWERED IN RESPONSE TO ABOVE QUESTION
      b.   (PALLIATIVE BEHAVIOR) Did you do anything to DEAL
           WITH your feelings of (as above)?

IF YES,

  c. WHAT? (Specify)

  d. HOW OFTEN did you do this? (all the time, most of the time sometimes, rarely, never)

  e. How did you feel THEN? (Specify)

IF NO,

  f. Did you just WAIT for it to go away, OR did you DO SOME-THING to work it out? (Wait, did something)

IF "DO SOMETHING",

  g. WHAT? (Specify)

  h. How OFTEN? (all the time, most of the time, sometimes, rarely, never)

  i. How did you feel THEN? (Specify)

IF ANY ANSWER EXCEPT "WAIT FOR IT TO GO AWAY"

  j. Did you ever do ANYTHING ELSE to make yourself feel better? (Yes, No)

IF YES,

  k. What? (Specify)

  l. How OFTEN? (all the time, most of the time, sometimes, rarely, never)

  m. How did you feel THEN? (Specify)

030. (SUBSTITUTE BEHAVIOR) Did you ever do anything to AVOID (problem) or to give yourself SOMETHING ELSE TO DO, so it wouldn't happen again? (Yes, No)

IF YES,

  a. WHAT? (Specify)

  b. HOW OFTEN? (all the time, most of the time, sometimes, rarely, never)

  c. When you did this, what happened NEXT? (Specify)

  d. Did you feel any DIFFERENT as a result? (Yes, No)

IF YES,

  e. WHAT was the change? (Specify)

IF NO, RESTATE:

  f. Did you ever try to KEEP YOURSELF BUSY, or to go somewhere else, to try to prevent the problem? (Yes, No)

IF YES,

  g. WHAT? (Specify)

  h. HOW OFTEN? (all the time, most of the time, sometimes, rarely, never)

  i. When you did this, what happened NEXT? (Specify)

  j. Did you feel any DIFFERENT as a result? (Yes, No)

IF YES,

  k. WHAT was the change? (Specify)

IF ANY ANSWER TO ABOVE QUESTIONS,

l. Did you ever do ANYTHING ELSE to keep yourself out of the problem situation? (Yes, No)

IF YES,

m. WHAT? (Specify)

n. HOW OFTEN? (all the time, most of the time, sometimes, rarely, never)

o. When you did this, what happened NEXT? (Specify)

p. Did you feel any DIFFERENT as a result? (Yes, No)

IF YES,

q. WHAT was the change? (Specify)

031. (PROBLEM-SOLVING BEHAVIOR) Did you ever do anything to try to SOLVE or IMPROVE the situation? (Yes, No)

IF YES,

a. WHAT? (Specify)

b. HOW OFTEN? (all the time, most of the time, sometimes, rarely, never)

c. What was the RESULT? (Specify)

d. How did you FEEL about that? (Specify)

IF NO, RESTATE:

e. Did you ever do anything to CHANGE things or to change yourself so that the problem would be better? (Yes, No)

IF YES,

f. WHAT? (Specify)

g. HOW OFTEN? (all the time, most of the time, sometimes, rarely, never)

h. What was the RESULT? (Specify)

i. How did you FEEL about that? (Specify)

IF ANY ANSWER TO ABOVE,

j. Did you ever do ANYTHING ELSE to try to solve the problem or to change the situation? (Yes, No)

IF YES,

k. WHAT? (Specify)

l. HOW OFTEN? (all the time, most of the time, sometimes, rarely, never)

m. What was the RESULT? (Specify)

n. How did you FEEL about this? (Specify)

032. Was there anything ELSE you did when the problem occurred, something we haven't mentioned before? (Yes, No)

IF YES,

a. WHAT? (Specify)

b. HOW OFTEN? (all the time, most of the time, sometimes, rarely never)

    c. What was the RESULT? (Specify)
    d. How did that make you FEEL? (Specify)

033. Looking back on the problem now, what do you think would have been the best way to deal with it? (Specify)

[Questions 34–45 repeat 28–33 for second and third problems.]

Now I have a few other general questions about your life on the outside.

046. How much did you DAYDREAM or fantasize? (all the time, most of the time, sometimes, rarely, never)
    a. When you did daydream, what was it mostly ABOUT? (Specify)
    b. In your daydreams, did you imagine a DIFFERENT life? (Yes, No)
    IF YES,
    c. WHAT things were changed? (Specify)

047. How much did you think of your CURRENT SITUATION, your life at that time? (all the time, most of the time, sometimes, rarely, never)
    a. Were you PLANNING your time or living day by day? (Plan, day × day)

048. How often did you think about the future? (all the time, most of the time, sometimes, rarely, never)
    a. Did you have definite plans or ideas about the FUTURE? (Yes, No)
    IF YES
    b. What? (Specify)
    c. How often did you think about the past? (all the time, most of the time, sometimes, rarely, never)

049. In general, were you SATISFIED with your life on the outside? (Yes, No)
    a. What CHANGES would have made your life better? (Specify)
    b. Did you ever TRY to make these changes? (Yes, No)

050. On the average, how often did you feel DEPRESSED? (__/week)
    a. On the average, how often did you feel ANGRY? (__/week)
    b. On the average, how often did you feel ANXIOUS? (__/week)
    c. On the average, how often did you feel GUILTY? (__/week)

All right, we've talked about your life generally, but how about the circumstances of your offense? We would like to know whether there was any relation between your offense and the problems you faced.

051. Were you arrested for a SINGLE offense or a SERIES of offenses? (Single, series)

(IF SERIES, the following questions will normally refer to the first offense of the series; this should be specified to the inmate. However, check also the circumstances of the last offense before arrest, whether the nature of the offenses changed over time, and whether unusual or emotional coping behavior developed during the sequence.)

052. Had anything UNUSUAL happened in the period just BEFORE your offense? (Yes, No)
     IF YES,
     a.   Please DESCRIBE the unusual events. (Specify)

053. Had any of the PROBLEMS we just discussed happened just before your offense? (Yes, No)
     IF YES,
     a.   WHICH? (Specify)

054. Were you FEELING angry, tense or depressed just before the offense? (Yes, No)
     IF YES,
     a.   WHICH? (Angry, depressed, tense)
     IF NO,
     b.   How did you feel? (Specify)

055. Were you drinking or using DRUGS just before the offense? (Yes, No)
     IF YES,
     a.   WHAT drugs? (Specify)
     b.   HOW MUCH? (__ total dosage)

056. Do you think there was any CONNECTION between the offense and the way you were dealing with things? (Yes, No)
     IF YES,
     a.   WHAT was the connection? (Specify)

057. Have you got any idea about which institution you'll be going to from here? (Yes, No)
     IF YES,
     a.   Where? (Specify)
     b.   Where would you like to go if you had the choice? (Specify)
     c.   What kinds of advantages or good things can you see in going to this institution? (Specify)
     d.   What kinds of problems? (Specify)

PART C. LIFE IN PRISON

Now I want to talk about your life IN PRISON. Everybody has some problems here just as on the outside. We would like to know about these problems and how you deal with them. As well, there are some things that you may like here, or that you may feel are helpful to you, and we would like to know about these too. First, let's look at how you plan to spend your time in prison.

001. How much time do (will) you SLEEP? (__ hours/day)

002. Do you have any PROBLEMS sleeping? (Yes, No)
    IF YES,
    a. WHAT? (Elucidate symptoms and reasons if possible; distinguish especially getting to sleep from early waking.)
    b. Do you use any DRUGS to help you sleep? (Yes, No)
    c. Do you ever sleep during the DAY? (Yes, No)
    IF YES,
    d. Would you describe this as NAPPING or longer sleep periods? (napping, longer (average hours __/day)

003. Do you WANT a job or to get into an educational or training program? (Yes, No)
    IF YES,
    a. WHAT job or program do you want?
       (Specify _____)
    b. What do you expect to get out of this job (program)?
       (Specify)

004. Aside from sleeping, how much time in the average week do (will) you spend on:
    a. WORK, school or training program (__ hours/week)
    b. VISITS and writing letters (__ hours/week)
    c. With FRIENDS, socializing (__ hours/week)
    d. Group MEETINGS (__ hours/week)
    e. Watching TV, listening to radio or music (__ hours/week)
    f. SPORTS and hobbies (__ hours/week)
    g. OTHER things (__ hours/week)
    (If more than 3 hours/week in categories d, e, f, or g then specify.)

005. Some of the time you have a choice of whether you will stay in your CELL or go onto the range. Of this time, what percentage do you spend in your cell?
    IF >0,
    a. WHY do you stay in your cell rather than on the range? (Specify)
    b. Does your cell time INCREASE OR DECREASE when you're have a problem? (Increase, decrease, same)
    IF INCREASE,
    c. Is this BECAUSE you stay in your cell to avoid problems? (Yes, No)
    IF YES
    d. How does it help? (Specify)

IF DECREASE
   e. Is this because it's easier to deal with problems when you're out of your cell? (Yes, No)
   IF YES
   f. How does it help? (Specify)

006. Do you have any close FRIENDS here?
   IF YES,
   a. How MANY? (# __)
   b. Where did you MEET them? (Here, previous prison term, outside)
   c. How would you best describe the way you socialize with other inmates here
     (i)   Pretty much on my own
     (ii) With a few close friends
     (iii) Part of a larger group (specify if possible)
     (iv) Float around, with lots of friends and acquaintances
     (v) Other
   d. Why do you choose to do your time that way? (Specify)

007. While you are in prison:
   a. WHO does (do you expect to) WRITE to you? (List)
   b. HOW MANY letters do you (expect to) get? (__/week or __ month)
   c. How many letters would you LIKE to get? (__/week or __ month)
   If discrepancy:
   d. Why do you want more/less?
   e. Who do you (are you going to) WRITE TO? (List)
   f. HOW MANY letters do you (plan to) write? (__/week or __ month)

008. Who visits (do you EXPECT will VISIT) you? (List)
   a. HOW MANY visits do you get (expect)? (__/week or __ month)
   b. How many visits would you like? (__/week or __ month)
   If discrepancy:
   c. Why do you want more/less?

009. Do you have any general PLAN as to how you are going to do your time? (Yes, No)
   a. What is the BEST WAY to do time? (Specify)
   b. Do you PLAN your time or live DAY BY DAY? (Plan, Day × Day)
   c. Is there anything that you want to ACCOMPLISH here, for example something you want to learn or changes you want to make in yourself? (Yes, No)
   IF YES,
   d. WHAT? (Specify)

e. Which of the following would best describe the way you (plan to) live here?
   (i)   Avoid trouble, keep busy and do what's necessary to get out as soon as possible
   (ii) Do something to improve or better myself while I'm in here
   (iii) Forget the outside, learn how to operate in the institution and have as good a time as possible here

Now I'd like to talk about PROBLEMS you are experiencing here.

010. Could you tell me what are the major PROBLEMS you have (expect to have) here? (Specify)

(In discussion below, problem areas enumerated here may be omitted.)

I. External

Now there are a wide variety of things that people find difficult about prison. Some of them are the things you have mentioned, but there are others that may have been left out. I would like to go over these with you just to make sure that we get a good picture of the problems you are facing. The first set of problems deals with things about the PHYSICAL environment in prison. That is, things around you that you see every day. For example, you may be bothered about things in the building here. It may be too hot or too cold or dirty or something else.

011. Do things about the BUILDING bother you? (Yes, No)
     IF YES,
     a. WHAT? (Specify)

012. Aside from the place, what about the LIVING ARRANGEMENTS? Do you have any problems in this area? (Yes, no)
     IF YES,
     a. WHAT?
     IF NO,
     b. Some common complaints we get are about the lack of PRIVACY, and CROWDING. Do things of this sort bother you? (Yes, No)
     IF YES,
     c. WHAT is the problem? (Specify)

013. What about the SERVICES and activities? Do you have any problems in this area? (Yes, no)
     IF YES
     a. WHAT? (Specify)
     IF FOLLOWING AREAS NOT ALL COVERED BY ABOVE ANSWER, ASK:
     a. This includes FOOD. Is the food a problem for you?

IF YES

b. Why? (Specify)

c. Are there any problems for you with MEDICAL SERVICES? (Yes, no)

IF YES

What? (Specify)

d. This area includes EDUCATIONAL AND VOCATIONAL TRAINING. Any problems there? (Yes, no)

IF YES

What? (Specify)

e. What CHANGES in any of these services would make your life better here?

014. Other than people, what are the THINGS about the outside that YOU MISS most here? (List up to 5 things (RANK ORDER))
What are some other things you WOULD LIKE TO HAVE that you don't have here now?

015. How often are you BORED? (__/week)

a. Is this a PROBLEM? (Yes, No)

016. Aside from the physical setup here do you have any problems with the RULES or procedures here? (Yes, No)

IF YES,

a. WHAT? (Specify)

THE FOLLOWING MAY BE OMITTED IF COVERED IN ABOVE ANSWER

b. Sometimes guys feel that there is a problem because the rules are enforced INCONSISTENTLY. Is this a problem for you? (Yes, No)

c. Do you feel that you KNOW THE SYSTEM here well enough to avoid getting into trouble? (Yes, No)

II. Interpersonal

Now we've covered the external environment; next I'd like to talk about how you get along with other inmates.

017. What kinds of problems do you have with OTHER INMATES? Do you find you have any difficulties fitting in or getting along with other inmates?

IF NONE,

a. Some guys find other inmates too AGGRESSIVE, or sometimes the opposite, that they're whining and BOTHERSOME. Do any of these things bother you? (Yes, no)

IF YES

HOW? (Specify)

b. I don't want any names but, are there any PARTICULAR IN-MATES who cause you problems or who you expect will cause you problems? (Yes, no)

IF YES

c. WHY (Specify)

d. Is there any particular SITUATION with other inmates which causes you problems? (Yes, no)

IF YES

e. WHAT? (Specify)

f. What about physical SAFETY. Do you feel in any danger here? (Yes, no)

IF YES

g. WHY? (Specify)

018. Do you have any problems or expect to have any problems with correctional officers or GUARDS?

IF YES

a. DESCRIBE the problem(s). (Specify)

019. What about OTHER STAFF, for example, CLASSIFICATION OFFICERS, or program staff; do you have any problems there? (Yes, No)

IF YES

a. WHAT? (Specify)

b. How often are they helpful to you? (all the time, most of the time, sometimes, rarely, never)

c. What could they do to be more helpful to you? (Specify)

020. What about problems with people not here, that is, people on the OUTSIDE? Who are the people you miss most here? (List)

a. How often do you THINK OF SOMEONE on the outside that you miss? (all the time, most of the time, sometimes, rarely, never)

b. Does thinking of people on the outside make it easier or harder for you? (acceptable: no difference)

III. Internal

Finally let's talk about thoughts that bother you, things inside yourself.

021. What sorts of problems do you have with THOUGHTS? (Specify)

IF NONE,

a. Well, many guys keep remembering things about their PAST and this upsets them. Does this ever happen to you? (Yes, no)

IF YES,

WHAT? (Specify)

IF No,

b. Some guys remember things they've DONE and feel they've messed up their lives or remember pleasant experiences and miss them. Do you do this? (Yes, no)

IF YES

c. Describe what you think.

d. What about thoughts of the PRESENT, for example, missing people you care for, or thinking that you are wasting your life, or any other thoughts you have about your life now. Would you tell me what thoughts you have about your life now? (Specify)

e. What thoughts do you have about the FUTURE? (Specify)

IF NONE,

f. FOR EXAMPLE you might worry about becoming institutionalized or that you might have big problems when you get out, or that you might be coming back to prison after you get out?

Do you ever think about things like this? (Yes, no)

IF YES,

g. What? (Specify)

h. Do you try to think about things here, do you try NOT to think about things, or do you just let things happen?

022. Are there any OTHER problems that come to mind, problems that we've left out? (Yes, No)

IF YES,

a. WHAT? (Specify)

Now that we have a list of your problems here, we would like to see which are the most important ones. First, I'll go over the problems I've noted. (Read)

023. Of the things we've discussed, could you tell me which are the MOST IMPORTANT? Rank order them. (Up to $n=5$)

Rank. . . . . .Item. . . . .

1.

2.

3.

4.

5.

If HE CAN'T RANK USE PAIRWISE COMPARISONS TO CONSTRUCT ORDER

024. When you have a problem, who are you likely to turn to for HELP? (Self, spouse, family, friend, professional) (Specify)

IF "IT DEPENDS" (give highest ranked problem as example)

COPING ANALYSIS

(From the problems listed above, three should be chosen if possible; an absolute minimum of two is required. Problems chosen should be in different areas, for which it is likely that different emotional responses are involved. Choose the highest ranked problems meeting these requirements.)

Now we'd like to talk about what you do when some of these problems occur

025. When __ (first problem) occurs, how does it make you FEEL? (Specify)
    IF NO CLEAR ANSWER,
    a. Do you feel ANGRY? (Yes, No)
    b. Do you feel DEPRESSED or low? (Yes, No)
    c. Do you feel ANXIOUS or uptight? (Yes, No)
    d. Do you feel GUILTY or ashamed? (Yes, No)
    IF MORE THAN ONE,
    e. Which do you feel MORE of? (Specify)

026. (DIRECT ACTION) When this happens, and you feel that way, WHAT DO YOU DO right then? (Specify)
    a. What happens THEN? (Specify)

    OMIT PARTS OF THE FOLLOWING SEQUENCES WHICH ARE ANSWERED IN RESPONSE TO ABOVE QUESTION
    a. (PALLIATIVE BEHAVIOR) Do you do anything to DEAL WITH your feelings of (as above)?
    IF YES,
    b. WHAT? (Specify)
    c. HOW OFTEN do you do this? (all the time, most of the time, sometimes, rarely, never)
    d. How do you feel THEN? (Specify)
    IF NO,
    e. Do you just WAIT for it to go away, OR do you DO SOMETHING to work it out? (Wait, do something)

    IF "DO SOMETHING,"
    f. WHAT? (Specify)
    g. How OFTEN? (all the time, most of the time, sometimes, rarely, never)
    h. How do you feel THEN? (Specify)
    IF ANY ANSWER EXCEPT "WAIT FOR IT TO GO AWAY"
    i. Do you ever do ANYTHING ELSE to make yourself feel better? (Yes, No)
    IF YES,
    j. What? (Specify)

    k. How OFTEN? (all the time, most of the time, sometimes, rarely, never)

    l. How do you feel after you do it? (Specify)

027. (SUBSTITUTE BEHAVIOR) Do you ever do anything to AVOID (problem) or to give yourself SOMETHING ELSE TO DO, so it won't happen again? (Yes, No)
IF YES,

    a. WHAT? (Specify)

    b. HOW OFTEN? (all the time, most of the time, sometimes, rarely, never)

    c. When you do this, what happens NEXT? (Specify)

    d. Do you feel any DIFFERENT as a result? (Yes, No)
IF YES,

    e. WHAT is the change? (Specify)
IF NO, RESTATE:

    f. Do you ever try to KEEP YOURSELF BUSY, or to go somewhere else, to try to prevent the problem? (Yes, No)
IF YES,

    g. WHAT? (Specify)

    h. HOW OFTEN? (all the time, most of the time, sometimes, rarely, never)

    i. When you do this, what happens NEXT? (Specify)

    j. Do you feel any DIFFERENT as a result? (Yes, No)
IF YES,

    k. WHAT is the change? (Specify)
IF ANY ANSWER TO ABOVE QUESTIONS,

    l. Do you ever do ANYTHING ELSE to keep yourself out of the problem situation? (Yes, No)
IF YES,

    m. WHAT? (Specify

    n. When you do this, what happens NEXT? (Specify)

    o. HOW OFTEN? (all the time, most of the time, sometimes, rarely, never)

    p. Do you feel any DIFFERENT as a result? (Yes, No)
IF YES,

    q. WHAT is the change? (Specify)

028. (PROBLEM-SOLVING BEHAVIOR) Do you ever do anything to try to SOLVE or IMPROVE the situation? (Yes, No)
IF YES,

    a. WHAT? (Specify)

    b. HOW OFTEN? (all the time, most of the time, sometimes, rarely, never)

    c. What is the RESULT? (Specify)

    d. How do you FEEL about that? (Specify)

    IF NO, RESTATE:

    e. Do you ever do anything to CHANGE things or to change your-self to try to solve the problem? (Yes, no)

    IF YES,

    f. WHAT? (Specify)

    g. HOW OFTEN? (all the time, most of the time, sometimes, rarely, never)

    h. What is the RESULT? (Specify)

    i. How do you FEEL about that (Specify)

    IF ANY ANSWER TO ABOVE,

    j. Do you ever do ANYTHING ELSE to try to solve the problem or to change the situation? (Yes, No)

    IF YES,

    k. WHAT? (Specify)

    l. HOW OFTEN? (all the time, most of the time, sometimes, rarely, never)

    m. What is the RESULT? (Specify)

    n. How do you FEEL about this? (Specify)

029. Is there anything ELSE you do when a problem occurs, something we haven't mentioned before? (Yes, No)

    IF YES,

    a. WHAT? (Specify)

    b. HOW OFTEN? (all the time, most of the time, sometimes, rarely, never)

    c. What is the RESULT? (Specify)

    d. How does that make you FEEL? (Specify)

Well, we've covered that problem pretty well. Let's turn to another and see what you do when IT happens.

[Questions 30–39 repeat 25–29 for second and third problems.]

040. a. On the average, how often do you feel ANGRY? (__/week)

    b. On the average, how often do you feel DEPRESSED? (__/week)

    c. On the average, how often do you feel ANXIOUS? (__/week)

    d. On the average, how often do you feel GUILT OR SHAME? (__/week)

We've been concentrating on your problems here. Let's look at the other side a little.

041. How often do you DAYDREAM? (all the time, most of the time, sometimes, rarely, never)

a. What ABOUT? (Specify)

b. Do you ever daydream that your life is DIFFERENT than what it is now? (Yes, No)

IF YES

c. How is it different? (Specify)

d. Do you ever imagine that you HADN'T BEEN CAUGHT? (Yes, no)

e. Do you tend to daydream MORE or LESS when you are faced with a difficult problem? (More, Less, Same)

IF NO DAYDREAM

f. What do you think about BEFORE YOU FALL ASLEEP at night? (Specify)

042. Do you KEEP IN TOUCH with current events? (Yes, No)

a. How often do you LISTEN TO NEWS on the radio or TV? (__/ week)

b. How often do you READ newspapers or news-magazines? (__/ week)

c. Do you try to keep in touch (not keep in touch) because you feel it makes it easier for you in here? (Yes, No)

043. Let's talk about some positive things here.

a. What are the things you consider HELPFUL to you? (Specify)

b. What are the good things about this place, things that you LIKE? (Specify)

c. What changes would make your life easier here? (Specify)

044. In general, how would you describe your life here? RATE how good it is on a scale where 100 is "all you would ever want from life" and 0 is "unbearable."

(Rating _____)

045. What plans do you have for the future? (Specify)

a. How often do you think about the future? (all the time, most of the time, sometimes, rarely, never)

b. How often do you think about the PAST? (all the time, most of the time, sometimes, rarely, never)

046. Is there anything you want to add which you consider important?

IF NO,

a. Is there anything else about life outside, or in prison, or the way you deal with problems that we haven't asked?

(Explain about being called back in future for questionnaires.)

Thank you!

END. THIS VERSION AS OF 16 MARCH 1980

Prison Control Scale

This questionnaire asks you to judge *how much control or influence* you think you have over some of the things which may happen to you *while in prison*. An example of something where you would have no control would be, let's say, the kind of hand you got in a poker game since this is pretty much determined by chance. On the other hand, you could have a lot of control over whether you win the hand or not since you could, for example, use your skills in bluffing or calculating odds. For each of the things listed below, could you please decide *how much control* or influence you think you have *while you're in prison*. Use a *number from 0 to 4* to give your answer where:

0 = is no control at all
1 = is very little control
2 = is some control
3 = is quite a bit of control
4 = is complete or total control

no control at all	very little control	some control	quite a bit of control	complete or total control
0	1	2	3	4

1. How often the people you love visit and write to you —
2. Getting your C.O. to support you for T.A.'s or parole —
3. Whether or not other inmates are friendly with you —
4. Whether you're punished in disciplinary court for an offense you didn't commit —
5. Getting a work change that you want —
6. Keeping yourself from getting frustrated or angry —
7. Staying in touch with the world and current events —
8. Not becoming institutionalized —
9. Getting to see your C.O. when you need to —
10. Whether your friends on the outside keep in touch with you —
11. Whether or not you get into arguments or hassles with security staff —
12. Being elected for the inmate committee —
13. Getting a transfer to a better institution —
14. How soon you get out of prison —
15. Keeping yourself from getting down and depressed —
16. Getting things set up for your release —
17. Getting help from staff when you need it —
18. Whether you end up in segregation —
19. Getting a cell change or range change when you want one —
20. Whether other inmates like or respect you —

no control at all	very little control	some control	quite a bit of control	complete or total control
0	1	2	3	4

21. Staying fit —
22. Solving family problems that may come up —
23. Keeping yourself from getting uptight and anxious —
24. Staying out of trouble in the institution —
25. Getting a phone call in an emergency —
26. Cheering up a friend who seems down and out —
27. Getting the guy in the cell next to yours to cut down the noise he — makes at night
28. Getting a shop instructor or teacher to help you with a problem —
29. Saying no to some good dope or brew —
30. Whether other inmates joke around and bug you —
31. Keeping yourself from getting lonely —
32. Staying on top of things in the institution —
33. Not losing your self-confidence —
34. Whether you end up doing something useful with your time in — prison
35. Getting problems with your canteen worked out —
36. Changing a bad habit you may want to change —
37. Changing your way of thinking about certain things while in — prison
38. Getting the doctor to give you medication when you feel you — need it
39. Working out an argument or misunderstanding you're having — with your wife or lady
40. Getting the institution to do something about a complaint or — grievance you have

TABLE A3. Summary of item–scale analysis for Prison Control scale.

Item number	M	SD	Item–scale Correlation
1.	2.13	1.17	.43
2.	2.15	1.15	.45
3.	2.93	0.80	.27
4.	1.22	1.28	.22
5.	2.72	1.01	.52
6.	3.01	0.93	.46
7.	3.32	0.89	.41
8.	3.18	1.19	.26
9.	2.95	0.87	.21
10.	1.95	1.25	.56
11.	2.81	1.05	.48
12.	2.37	1.34	.38
13.	1.95	1.14	.42
14.	2.13	1.25	.36
15.	3.00	1.01	.64
16.	3.15	0.94	.59
17.	2.20	1.12	.60
18.	2.58	1.43	.34
19.	2.07	1.31	.42
20.	2.87	0.81	.51
21.	3.40	0.76	.19
22.	2.30	0.94	.47
23.	2.98	0.89	.68
24.	3.17	0.96	.37
25.	2.97	0.96	.48
26.	3.00	0.92	.16
27.	2.95	1.10	.54
28.	3.07	0.82	.51
29.	3.13	1.28	.50
30.	2.82	1.03	.42
31.	2.58	1.06	.44
32.	3.02	0.89	.47
33.	3.15	0.95	.59
34.	3.43	0.79	.44
35.	3.05	0.98	.52
36.	2.82	1.07	.42
37.	3.05	0.95	.47
38.	1.75	1.28	.26
39.	2.68	1.03	.42
40.	1.95	1.13	.49
Total Scale	107.97	19.85	

Coefficient Alpha = .91

Note. Scores on each item could range from 0 to 4. Corrections for part-whole overlap were applied in calculating item–total scale correlations.

Prison Problems Scale

Listed below are some things that inmates often say bother them while doing time. For each item, could you please indicate how much it bothers you or how much of a problem it is for you personally. Use a number from 0 to 4 to give your answer where:

0 = doesn't bother you at all; never on your mind
1 = bothers you a little; rarely on your mind
2 = bothers you sometimes; sometimes on your mind
3 = bothers you a lot; often on your mind
4 = bothers you all the time; always on your mind

Not at all	a little	sometimes	a lot	all the time
0	1	2	3	4

1. Not knowing where you stand regarding T.A.'s, parole, etc. ___
2. Not fitting in with other inmates, nothing in common ___
3. Being bored, lots of idle time ___
4. Feeling out of touch with the world ___
5. Feeling guilty for your offense ___
6. Feeling angry with yourself ___
7. Afraid of returning to prison ___
8. Not being able to make decisions about your life ___
9. Not feeling physically safe ___
10. Missing social life and partying ___
11. Longing for a time in the past ___
12. Being told what to do ___
13. Not knowing the rules or having the rules changed ___
14. Feeling rotten for having been a criminal and messing up your life ___
15. Feeling angry with the world ___
16. Not being able to keep yourself out of trouble in the institution ___
17. Getting annoyed or irritated with other inmates ___
18. Staff out to make things difficult for you ___
19. Being apathetic, no motivation ___
20. Staff who don't care how you feel ___
21. Missing little "luxuries," e.g., your favorite food, your own clothes ___
22. Feeling sorry for yourself ___
23. Wishing that time would go faster ___
24. Afraid of losing your control ___
25. Feeling that your life has been wasted ___
26. Programs that don't help enough ___

Not at all	a little	sometimes	a lot	all the time
0	1	2	3	4

27. Family who forget you —
28. Wishing you had more privacy and quiet —
29. Not being able to run your life —
30. Feeling sexually frustrated —
31. Worrying about how you will cope when you get out —
32. Having no goals and ambitions —
33. Feeling hopeless —
34. No friends you can be close to —
35. Staff not listening to grievances —
36. Feeling worried about becoming institutionalized —
37. Being afraid of going crazy —
38. Losing self-confidence —
39. Feeling that you are unjustly being punished —
40. Missing somebody —

TABLE A4. Summary of item–scale analysis for Prison Problems scale.

Item number	M	SD	Item–scale Correlation
1.	2.02	1.26	.38
2.	0.85	1.10	.42
3.	1.40	1.21	.64
4.	1.47	1.32	.67
5.	0.73	1.15	.34
6.	1.18	1.24	.63
7.	1.51	1.56	.33
8.	1.45	1.35	.57
9.	0.50	0.91	.42
10.	2.58	1.24	.45
11.	1.77	1.50	.52
12.	2.10	1.34	.37
13.	1.07	1.06	.39
14.	1.23	1.33	.44
15.	0.62	0.98	.41
16.	0.58	0.98	.31
17.	1.63	1.09	.50
18.	1.00	1.16	.35
19.	1.00	1.04	.44
20.	0.83	1.15	.30
21.	2.85	1.13	.60
22.	0.57	0.98	.59
23.	2.63	1.53	.64
24.	1.28	1.24	.66
25.	1.40	1.33	.50
26.	1.48	1.37	.56
27.	1.30	1.45	.49
28.	2.43	1.39	.64
29.	2.73	1.51	.73
30.	2.60	1.24	.45
31.	1.67	1.46	.68
32.	0.77	1.12	.35
33.	0.80	1.21	.73
34.	0.95	1.32	.65
35.	0.96	1.25	.37
36.	0.80	1.19	.31
37.	0.58	1.06	.48
38.	0.67	1.13	.57
39.	1.38	1.50	.27
40.	3.25	0.95	.61
Total Scale	56.65	26.26	
Coefficient Alpha = .93			

Note. Scores on each item could range from 0 to 4. Corrections for part–whole overlap were applied in calculating item–total scale correlations.

Author Index

Subject Index